Eating
Well for
Menopause

Dr Laura Wyness and Lynn Burns

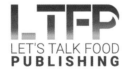

LET'S TALK FOOD
PUBLISHING

"Nothing prepares you for menopause, but resources like this are very reassuring because you know everything has been researched and tested. The book has been incredibly helpful for me, helping with balancing my eating and finding what works to reduce symptoms during this new phase of my life. It's very easy to follow, with a nice writing style. You have a way of making things seem so clear and easy for us non-scientists to understand."
Sasha Macsween

"The book is framed around women's personal experiences of menopause and what they want to know. It's based on science and is a highly accessible, relevant and informative book that all women, who want to look after their health as their bodies change, should read."
Claire Bell

"Whilst menopause is a natural stage in life, it can be an extremely confusing and overwhelming time to cope with. Nutrition is just one part of the menopause jigsaw, but it's a key area that can really have an impact on symptoms. This book is a wonderful guide to help with navigating through menopause and offering a way to gain control of at least one part of the puzzle. Easy to follow with really practical tips and delicious recipes. I wouldn't hesitate to recommend it as a genuine menopause must have."
Hazel Barton, Pharmacist and Menopause Champion

"I know this book will help so many people understand what's going on in their body and help them to take the right steps to deal with their menopause journey."
Yvonne Currie

"Sometimes it can be hard to cut through all the misinformation about nutrition on the internet which is all the more reason this book stands out. Written by two qualified and experienced Registered Nutritionists, Lynn and Laura have created a well-researched yet accessible book to help women understand what menopause is all about and the actions they can undertake to future-proof their health. It's a fantastic resource."
Dr Yvonne Finnegan (Nutrition Consultant and CORU Registered Dietitian)

"Loved it! A brilliant, well-researched and informative book with inspiring healthy recipes."
Brenda McPherson

This book is a great resource for women around the time of menopause, and for clinicians who are trying to help! It is extremely well-written and easy to read but is full of well-researched and evidenced information. I will add it to my list of go-to publications to which I signpost women when they are navigating some very confusing times.
Dr Rosie Cochrane, Consultant in Gynaecology and Sexual Health

"As a nutritionist who supports women experiencing menopause in the workplace, I'm always on the lookout for resources that provide accurate, evidence-based information. This book explains the science behind menopause by answering the questions that menopausal women ask, alongside practical tips and information and a dedicated recipe section to support eating well. It's a valuable resource for any woman wanting to make informed choices about their nutrition and health during this perfectly normal life stage."
Dr Emma Williams, Chair of Nutritionists in Industry, UK

"I have been working through the recipes. I am really enjoying them. The muffins went down well with the family. Very tasty low-sugar muffins that smell delicious when cooking. The salmon was a tasty quick and easy dinner. Great for mid-week! "
Anne Carter

"I obviously know about menopause having gone through it but this has given me a better understanding on how and why things happen as a result. I can't wait to try some of the recipes, especially if they can make a difference on how I feel!"
Shelly Burrows

"From women to women: a must-have book for those who want to alleviate these nasty menopause symptoms through a balanced diet."
Nathalie Tolchard

"Easy to read, science-based information and delicious recipes. I'd recommend this to anyone interested in learning more about eating well as they navigate through menopause."
Ruth Schofield

"What an amazing read. The pages include all of the information I have been searching for, all in one place. I like that the book explains, in detail, the science behind why certain foods and vitamins are good for us during the menopause but in a language that I can understand - whilst giving examples and alternatives of what to eat. It is also great to know why we may feel how we do, and have some healthy tips on how we can help our bodies and improve our lifestyle going forward."
Rosslyn Cooper

Published in 2023 by Let's Talk Food Publishing

Copyright © Dr Laura Wyness and Lynn Burns 2023

Dr Laura Wyness and Lynn Burns have asserted their right to be identified
as the authors of this Work in accordance with the
Copyright, Designs and Patents Act 1988

ISBN Paperback: 978-1-7393854-0-8
Ebook: 978-1-7393854-1-5

All rights reserved. No part of this publication may be reproduced, stored in a
retrieval system, or transmitted in any form or by any means, electronic,
mechanical, photocopying, recording or otherwise, without the prior permission of
the copyright owner.

A CIP catalogue copy of this book can be found in the British Library.

Published with the help of Indie Authors World
www.indieauthorsworld.com

Disclaimer

The information in this book is provided as an information resource only and is not to be used or relied on for any diagnostic, treatment or medical purpose. All health issues should be discussed with your GP and/or other qualified medical professional.

Although the authors have made every effort to ensure that the information in this book is correct at press time, the authors take no responsibility or liability for any loss, damage, claim or disruption caused by errors or omissions caused by any reason, not for any claim resulting from the use or misuse of the information provided.

The trademarks for Quorn are mentioned in this book, but this is not an endorsement by the Trademark owner.

Acknowledgements

This book is a product of many hands crafting it. Although we have both devoted many months researching, analysing recipes, writing and cooking, we have also had invaluable support and guidance.

Firstly, thank you to all the women who have asked us for nutritional advice and dietary support around menopause. Your questions have provided the inspiration for the structure and content of this book.

A mentoring chat with Jane Kearney helped us think about where we might like to go as a partnership. Thank you Jane for helping us structure our path to this point, that we had a book worth writing. We are hugely grateful for the confidence boost you gave us and for encouraging us to 'go for it!'

We are also extremely grateful for the mentorship from Ruth Clarke who has helped us think about our partnership which has supported our journey to where we are, and Joan Ransley from the Guild of Food Writers who helped nourish our initial thought that we could actually publish a proper book.

Thank you to our friend Gin Lalli, who shared her experience of successfully publishing her first book and for introducing us to Kim at Indie Authors. Kim and her wonderful team have made the process of publishing far less daunting. The Friday messages with inspirational quotes and gentle nudges were much appreciated!

Unlike many writers embarking on the book writing journey, we had the words. We 'just' needed to tweak them, 'only' do a bit of redrafting of our download pdf version. A good friend has often said to be very wary of the words 'just' and 'only'. John Broxis, how right you are! Thank you for your support and words of wisdom. The 'just' tweaking and 'only' a bit of redrafting has taken so much longer than we imagined to get us to the final manuscript.

Iain Wilson, thank you not only for the most amazing photos, but also for cooking and eating those recipes, so they were truly tested in every sense. Thanks also to Tessa Chaillou for advice on the cover design, your ideas and design ideas helped us to the final cover.

We must especially thank our respective husbands, Duncan and James, losing us to this project and supporting us all the way. Euan and Creagh being expert tasters and testers - growing teenage boys with appetites.

Thanks also to Sandy Cullen for general encouragement and sound advice and to Ilona, Maggie, Sasha and the 'Let's Talk Food' Facebook group members for feedback on recipes and drafts and kind words.

And finally, thank you to you for reading this book and supporting our work. Please keep talking about menopause.

Foreword

I am honoured to have the opportunity to write the foreword for Eating Well for Menopause by two highly respected Registered Nutritionists. As a public health nutritionist, I understand the important role that nutrition plays in our overall wellbeing, particularly during significant life transitions such as menopause.

Lynn and Laura are experts in their field, with years of experience. They have used their extensive knowledge and expertise to create an informative and practical guide to help women navigate the complex world of eating well for menopause.

Researching a healthy ageing diet is the area of my doctoral research. As we age, our bodies undergo significant changes and, for many women, menopause can be a challenging time. Menopausal symptoms can range from: hot flushes, weight gain and insomnia to brain fog, bladder issues and bone loss. They are issues that I regularly explore on my Women Positively Ageing podcast. We have the ability to influence the ageing process, but in order to live well for longer we need to make positive changes. The good news is that nutrition can play a vital role in mitigating menopausal symptoms and maintaining our health and wellbeing.

In this book, Lynn and Laura provide practical, easy-to-follow advice, along with a variety of very tasty recipes that will help women put the information contained in the book into practice.

What I love about this book is its down-to-earth focus on how to put what we know from science into practice. We eat food, not nutrients, so it's great that the book shares lots of food-related suggestions. Their approach is sensible and practical, making it easy for women to incorporate healthy eating habits into their daily routine.

Eating Well for Menopause is a fantastic resource for any woman looking to navigate the challenges of menopause. I highly recommend this book to anyone looking to make positive changes during this important life transition. With the help of the authors' expert guidance, you can eat well, feel well, and thrive during menopause and beyond.

Barbara Bray, MBE, FIFST, RNutr
Food Safety and Nutrition Consultant, PhD Researcher

Contents

Introduction

Welcome to *Eating Well for Menopause*, a book crafted from questions from women, asking how to eat better as they navigate menopause. We answer common questions about nutrition and menopause with science and simple food-based advice. To make this advice easier to put into practice we have supplemented it with recipes that anyone in the house will enjoy.

Menopause will come to all women, at different ages and in different ways. It is a time where many women focus on what they eat and how they live. Considering your diet can be so helpful in managing the common symptoms that affect most women to a greater or lesser extent. In addition, as menopause is a time where our bodies change, it is a good reminder to think more carefully about ageing with good health and quality of life.

Despite menopause being a part of women's lives, it has long been a taboo topic leaving women lacking good information and support. Clients were asking us about how to eat in a way to improve their menopause and it is their questions that have guided the writing of this book - the chapter titles reflect these questions that matter to women.

We were a little ahead of the media-led curve when we started our research on menopause. (Davina McCall had yet to share her story) but in the last few years, menopause is beginning to be talked about more openly. With this more open conversation, information on diet and nutrition is becoming more accessible and easier to find. However, some of it remains neither accurate nor helpful: whilst more sharing of experience can be positive and supportive, it can also be overwhelming and confusing, especially in the arena of dietary advice.

This is where *Eating Well for Menopause* comes in. It is a starting point, grounded in science, and, whilst nutrition is never black and white, the simple principles of this book will benefit most readers. We aim to share the nuance and where the science is still emerging. We hope this helps you to make informed decisions that work for you.

Our collaborative endeavours

Who would have thought that a quick virtual coffee would lead to a book? A virtual coffee before this became a normal thing, before the blip that was COVID. A nutritionist in Edinburgh reaching out to a nutritionist in France, to talk about freelance life and maybe help each other out.

There was something in the balance of our personalities and skill sets that worked. Both Registered Nutritionists, we love researching the science of nutrition and health, but we are also aware that people don't eat nutrients; they eat food. Talking about food can help make nutrition science more accessible and our aim now is to help translate the science into practical advice about food, dietary habits and of course tasty recipes! *'Let's Talk Food'* became the name for our collaborative endeavours.

Our main focus is to develop information resources and tailored recipes to support our clients. They were asking us about how the food they ate could actually help them through menopause. A pdf booklet answering their questions with a few downloadable recipes was the first step to where we are now.

The positive feedback we received showed us how valuable it was. People enjoyed the recipes and thanked us for the information. Groups of nutritionists wanted to know more and invited us to deliver some online talks. We developed an online course for health professionals to enhance the support to their menopausal clients. From this, the book was born.

Why you should read this book

The book outlines facts on diet and nutrition in relation to menopause, both with regard to symptoms and in aspects of health that change after menopause. We have structured the book in chapters that relate to the questions we have been asked by women seeking our advice.

We explain the science and talk about nutrients, then pull this together with practical food-based tips. Our aim is to inform and clarify how diet can help support women throughout peri-menopause and post-menopause.

With an increasing amount of information becoming available on all aspects of menopause beyond food and diet, we have included a list of links and resources from some trusted sources.

We have scattered bite-sized bits of information throughout, using some images to signpost you so that the book is easy to pick up and leaf through, as well as sit down and enjoy in a more in-depth way.

Look out for our:

Top Tips   **Did You Know?**   **The Science Says**

Extra tips to put information into action, surprising facts or a little extra detail about the science are highlighted. To make the information practical we have included some simple and delicious recipes. Food that appeals to anyone.

Throughout the recipe section we have also included some suggestions for adapting the recipes.

Look out for our:

Have You Tried?   **Easy Upgrades**

These highlight where we have included some quick tips and quick-make additions.

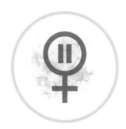

Menopause

A summary: When, how long it takes and the symptoms

Definition

The most simple way to define menopause is when menstruation comes to an end. Menopause is literally translated as 'periods stop'. This process affects women differently, according to the British Menopause Society, three quarters of menopausal women in the UK say that it has caused them to change their lives. (BMS, 2017)

When does it happen and how long does it take?

Menopause can occur naturally anywhere between 40 and 60 years. The average age in the UK is 51 years.

Although, scientifically speaking, menopause is defined as the last menstrual period, we generally use the term 'menopause' to describe the whole process of hormones changing through peri-menopause until a year after periods have ceased.

The transition through menopause is thought to be around 2-5 years. It is a very individual experience, menopause can happen quite suddenly (only a few months) for some. For others, it can happen over a few years. Some women report symptoms lasting for more than 5 years or diminishing to return a few years later.

Pre-Menopause	is the time between a women's first menstrual period and the onset of peri-menopause.
Peri-Menopause	is the time when your hormones start to change in preparation for menopause and periods become irregular or you may completely skip one or more periods. It includes the time from the onset of menopausal symptoms and the first year after menopause.
Menopause	is a point in time 12 months after the final menstrual period.
Post-Menopause	is the time after menopause, when a woman hasn't had a period for over a year. You will no longer have periods but some women may continue to experience symptoms of menopause.

Menopause can happen under 40 years of age, affecting around 1 in 100 women. Early menopause can run in families or be a side effect of some treatments, for example chemotherapy, or surgery to remove the ovaries.

As oestrogen provides some positive health effects, notably on heart and bone health, diet and lifestyle changes are important for all post-menopausal women but particularly so for women who reach menopause much earlier in life.

What does it feel like?

Menopausal symptoms can start a few years before your periods stop and can last for four or more years after your last period. Women report a wide range of symptoms and every woman will experience their own combination. Most people are aware of hot flushes (flashes) as a menopausal symptom as this is the most commonly experienced symptom.

Falling oestrogen has a role in all menopausal symptoms to a greater or lesser degree. In addition to menopause, other factors such as stress, ageing and lifestyle can exacerbate these symptoms or be responsible for them. Changes to diet and lifestyle can help manage many of the

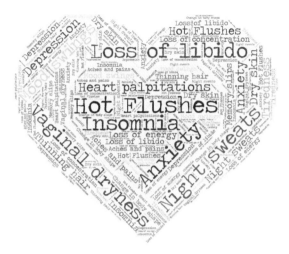

symptoms experienced during menopause and will no doubt help maintain health long after menopause. Even so, menopause can be challenging and many factors influence its symptoms, some you have little control over. Changing diet and lifestyle alone may be sufficient for some but certainly not for all. It is important to be kind to yourself and seek advice to help manage symptoms if you are struggling.

How does menopause affect my health and well-being?

The effects the drop in oestrogen has on health and how the body changes at this time of life affects everyone differently. Women have a wide range of questions and challenges. We have pulled together the most common questions that women ask about health and menopause to structure the chapters of the book. In the pages that follow, we give some answers and some practical lifestyle tips for these aspects of managing menopause:

- Hot flushes and night sweats make life uncomfortable – how much can lifestyle reduce them and lessen their effect?
- How can I best manage my weight during the menopause and maintain muscle?
- Heart health - now that I have hit menopause is my risk of heart disease much higher?

- How does menopause affect my bones? Am I at risk of osteoporosis?
- I read that depression and anxiety are more common during menopause. Can diet lessen the effects that menopause has on emotions and mood?
- Does menopause affect sleep and can my diet improve it?
- How can I stay well hydrated without going to the toilet all the time?
- Can diet stop menopausal hair loss and my skin becoming dry?
- Supplements and diets for menopause - do they deliver what they promise?
- Where can I find evidence based advice on managing menopause?
- How do I put this into practice in my kitchen?

More than just menopause

Some of these health issues are directly related to hormonal changes. For most questions, however, there are a combination of factors at play which can exacerbate or cause these health issues.

At this time in women's lives there can be a lot of changes - children growing up, changes in careers, older parents needing support etc. These situations can result in health issues independently of menopause. Equally, stress and other health issues can make menopausal symptoms feel more intense or exacerbate problems that are related to hormones.

Often, improvements in diet and lifestyle can have a significant positive effect on all of these things, not those solely related to the drop in oestrogen. Many of them benefit everyone in the household and can be achieved without adding stress or cost to the food provision.

This is also a time when many women really feel differently about their bodies. Noticing changes related to getting older and more mature can be a wake-up call that it is time to care more about ourselves, not just everyone around us. This should be harnessed to power the motivation to make positive change, investing in ourselves not only to ease menopausal symptoms but also to protect health and well-being into older age. We hope that the advice in this book will help you to do just that.

A note to non-binary and transgender readers

Menopause is a biological process affecting everyone born with ovaries and who experience menstruation however they express their gender or sexuality. Menopausal symptoms can affect anyone who experiences a drop or loss of female hormones circulating in their bodies. Changes to the levels of female hormones are important to your well-being and wider health. If you are experiencing symptoms associated with a reduction of oestrogen and progesterone in your body, it is important to talk openly with your GP. Since individual and person-centred care is so important, it is good to see that transgender and non-binary people are to be included in National Institute of Health and Care Excellence guidelines on menopause for the first time.

This book generally uses the terms 'women' and 'woman' with no intention of exclusion - simply the research and literature we have been learning from has been on evidence gathered on menopause in cis-women. Unfortunately, there is very little evidence specifically for transgender people on the effects of hormone changes so we are unable to give specific advice to this group.

However, much of the advice contained in this book is likely to be helpful with menopause like symptoms and health issues related to fluctuations in female hormones. The advice is also beneficial for healthy ageing and general health and well-being for everyone.

There is specific advice on menopause for transgender people from "The Menopause Management".(The Menopause Management, 2022)

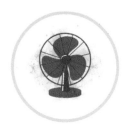

Hot Flushes

How diet can impact hot flushes?

Hot flushes or flashes are thought to affect about 80% of menopausal women, and it is the most commonly recognised symptom of menopause. (RockMyMenopause) What is going on? Whilst we think of oestrogen as a reproductive hormone, it actually affects organs around the body, including the hypothalamus in the brain which is responsible for regulating temperature. As oestrogen falls, the ability to regulate temperature gets glitchy.

For some women hot flushes and night sweats are a mild inconvenience easily managed by wearing layers or adjusting the environment accordingly. For others they can cause a lot of discomfort and inconvenience making work or sleep difficult. So while they can be thought of as a minor issue, the knock on effects this has on well-being through poor sleep or effects on concentration and productivity can be a real challenge.

If they are a challenge for you then do seek advice as they can persist for some time, maybe for years. They can also return months or years after you felt they had become a thing of the past. Everyone is different.

Can what we eat impact hot flushes?

It seems that what we eat can impact the intensity and frequency of hot flushes for some women – some foods have been shown to reduce these and other foods seem to act as triggers.

Soya can turn down the heat

Soya foods have been shown to be beneficial for managing hot flushes. Rich in plant compounds similar to oestrogen, known as isoflavones or phytoestrogens, soya foods appear to dampen down the effect of the drop in human oestrogen on the hypothalamus.

phytoestrogen

[fī'tō-ĕs'trə-jən]

(n.) Any of a group of substances, including isoflavones, that are derived from plants and have biological effects on animals similar to those of oestrogen.

Two servings of soya a day has been shown to reduce hot flushes to varying degrees in women. (Taku, 2012) There is limited evidence that the same effect is gained from phytoestrogen or isoflavone supplements. (see Myths and Marketing chapter)

It usually takes several weeks for the effects to be felt and it is advisable to increase the soya in your diet gradually. Too much too quickly can result in some bloating and discomfort.

There are other benefits from adding soya into the diet. Protein in soya seems to have a positive effect on heart health – see Heart Health chapter.

Five Ways to Enjoy Soya

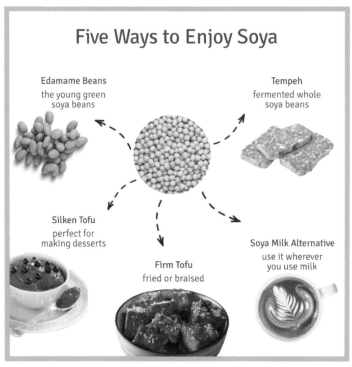

Edamame Beans
the young green
soya beans

Tempeh
fermented whole
soya beans

Silken Tofu
perfect for
making desserts

Firm Tofu
fried or braised

Soya Milk Alternative
use it wherever
you use milk

Soya: What is a serving?

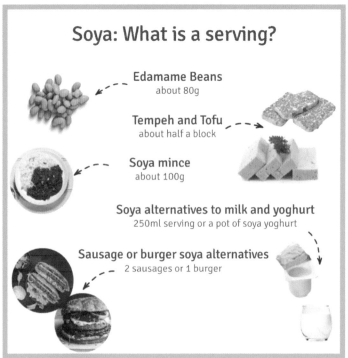

Edamame Beans
about 80g

Tempeh and Tofu
about half a block

Soya mince
about 100g

Soya alternatives to milk and yoghurt
250ml serving or a pot of soya yoghurt

Sausage or burger soya alternatives
2 sausages or 1 burger

Women often fear that consuming soya foods increase the risk of breast cancer. It is reassuring that leading global cancer organisations such as the World Cancer Research Fund (WCRF), the American Institute of Cancer Research (AICR), American Cancer Society (ACS), and the European Food Safety Authority all agree that soya foods are safe for women in relation to breast cancer, be that the risk of developing it, when living with breast cancer, or the risk of recurrence in those women who have been successfully treated. (Messina et al, 2022)

 Evidence from human studies in breast cancer patients consistently show that soya foods and drinks are safe and do not increase risk of breast cancer. It's perfectly safe for breast cancer survivors and those at high risk to include soya as part of a healthy balanced diet. There is some evidence that soya may actually help protect women against breast cancer.

Foods that can turn up the heat

Foods that some women find exacerbate hot flushes include spicy food, alcohol, caffeine and some cheeses. The evidence is not conclusive, however all of these foods have components that some people are sensitive to and may result in feeling a little flushed. This effect may be heightened in menopausal women to a greater or lesser degree.

One way to spot foods that may be problematic for you to is to keep a note – if you are hit by hot flushes that wake you at night or interfere with your day, reflect on the foods and drinks that you have eaten in the hour or so before hand.

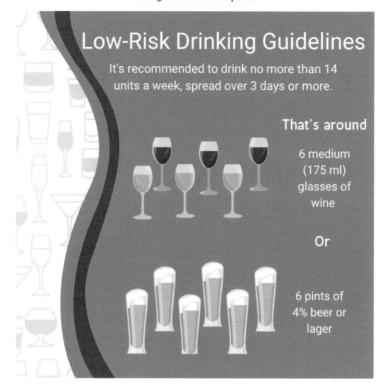

Low-Risk Drinking Guidelines

It's recommended to drink no more than 14 units a week, spread over 3 days or more.

That's around

6 medium (175 ml) glasses of wine

Or

6 pints of 4% beer or lager

Cheese has compounds in it that act a bit like adrenaline, the key one is called tyramine. Some people when they eat a lot of cheese break out in sweats or get headaches. It may explain why for some women, cheese can seem to trigger or amplify hot flushes or sweats during menopause.

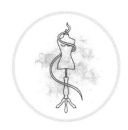

Healthy Weight Management

How can I best manage my weight during the menopause and maintain muscle?

Does menopause itself cause weight gain?

Many menopausal women worry about weight gain during menopause and looking on the internet it would seem that menopause causes dramatic weight gain. If we look at the evidence however, women, on average, gain approximately 2 to 3kg over the course of the menopause transition. There seems to be a wide variation around this average with some women gaining more and some who may not experience weight gain. (Marlatt et al. 2022)

As we get older, our lifestyle changes. Children, work pressures, lack of available time to cook and exercise can all contribute to how we eat and how active we are. Some of this can be associated with age and life just getting in the way of self-care. Menopausal symptoms can be part of this or exacerbate these things.

Weight management is much more complicated than often depicted in the media. It is affected by lots of factors including poor sleep, anxiety, fatigue, aches and pains and depression. These are all issues that are commonly reported by menopausal women and it is here where menopause can exert its effect on weight management.

While hormone changes of menopause do not seem to affect weight management directly, the symptoms and effects on women may impact weight management. By managing menopausal symptoms well, the effect they have on appetite and weight management can be lessened to some degree.

Focusing on positive lifestyle changes that are good for health and general weight management will be more effective than restrictive weight loss diets that may exacerbate menopausal symptoms.

Changes in body shape

How weight is carried can be affected by menopausal changes in oestrogen levels. Body fat can be redistributed. Many women find that their body shape changes, although everyone is different.

The change in shape may be due to oestrogen levels dropping and results in fat being carried in a way more similar to men, sitting more on the stomach and middle. During childbearing years fat tends to sit on the hips and thighs.

The way fat is distributed is important to health. Fat sitting on the stomach or middle seems to be more strongly associated with the risk of heart disease and type 2 diabetes. (Gibson & Ashwell, 2020)

This change in shape can affect self-confidence and body image for many women. It may also give the impression of gaining weight, leading to dieting that may lead to low intakes of nutrients important to managing health and menopausal symptoms.

Accepting that our body may change and in a way that might be beyond our control can be important to our mental and physical health. Gratitude for the body we have and that it deserves nourishment and movement to keep it healthy unconditionally can be a helpful mindset.

Unintentional weight loss is not healthy

Weight management is not just about weight gain. Losing weight unintentionally or too quickly can be a sign that you are not meeting your nutritional requirements.

It may mean that the weight lost is due to muscle loss which as we age is really important to avoid. We naturally start to lose muscle as we age so it is important not speed up this process.

Too little protein throughout the day results in protein from our muscles being used to meet our protein needs. This can affect our strength and fitness. Protein is also important for the strength of our bones and how well our immune system works. So, if we are losing weight, either by choice or unintentionally, we must guard against low protein intakes and losing muscle.

In accepting and caring for a changing body we must take care that it is well nourished. Being underweight or losing weight too fast by following a diet or eating pattern that cuts out many foods can affect the strength of our bones, our fitness, how easily we get ill and how long it takes us to recover.

Unintentional weight loss can also be an early sign of a health problem that needs treatment. Suddenly being able to wear a dress that hasn't fitted you for years without any attempt at losing weight should be questioned a little, not just celebrated.

Can menopause result in weight loss?

Whilst it is true that some symptoms of menopause can make it easier to gain weight, for some people the opposite can be true. Here are two examples:

Poor sleep

It is true that poor sleep can be associated with cravings for calorie rich, sometimes sweet foods. It is very personal but being aware of this can help to avoid weight gain. In addition, fatigue can lead us to be less motivated to be active, which can also contribute to weight gain.

On the other hand, poor sleep can have a negative effect on mood and, combined with fatigue, may reduce appetite. Combined with a lack of motivation to shop and cook, this can have the opposite effect and contribute to unintentional weight loss.

Anxiety and depression

Stress and low mood can lead to eating more frequently, being drawn to higher calorie foods, which can lead to weight gain. This can be exacerbated by a lack of motivation to self-care, exercise and cook well.

For others it can cause a loss of appetite and lack of interest in food. It can also lead to people moving more and being less able to sit calmly. This can contribute to unintentional weight loss.

Tips for healthy weight management

Don't skip meals

Skipping meals makes it harder to meet our nutritional requirements. If you are not so hungry then have a mini-meal, a snack that contains some protein and carbohydrates. It could be something like hummus and crackers, a small sandwich, toast and nut butter or mixture of nibbles that include dried fruit, nuts and a yoghurt.

If you are trying to lose weight, skipping meals can leave you feeling more tired, can affect your mood and restricts not only your calories but other vital nutrients. It can make you crave sweet and easy-to-grab high-energy but less nutritious foods.

It is better to space meals out across the day and adjust portion size to your appetite.

Include protein at every meal

Protein helps satisfy your hunger and may help reduce cravings, which can be very helpful in maintaining a healthy weight.

If we do need to, or want to lose weight, then it's important that we do not lose muscle mass in the process. Including adequate protein in your diet throughout the day and protein snacks after activity helps to prevent muscle loss when you lose weight. This is more important as we age because it's harder to build and regain muscle as we get older.

Although most people in the UK meet the recommended protein requirements, it's often not evenly spaced out across the day. Research from sports science has taught us that our muscles can use protein better if it's eaten across the day rather than concentrated in one or two main meals. (Mamerow et al, 2014) Our muscles seem to be able to use protein most effectively in the hours after activity. Eating a protein rich snack or meal soon after we have been active is a good practice.

Include plenty fruits and vegetables and fibre-rich foods

Including a variety of fruits, vegetables, oats, whole grain bread, brown rice, whole grain pasta, beans, peas and lentils will provide beneficial fibre to your diet. This helps us to feel satisfied for longer and also feeds our gut microbes.

A healthy gut microbiome, the diverse collection of microbes living in our colon, is involved with appetite regulation and healthy weight management. Including a variety of plant foods in your diet increases the diversity of your gut microbiome, and a diverse gut microbiome is associated with better overall health, not just better appetite control.

Mindful eating

Being aware of your internal body signals of hunger and fullness can help you tailor portions sizes to suit your needs.

Considering whether you are physically hungry, if you are craving food or want to eat in response to another emotion is a first step.

Mindful eating takes some practice and can help you determine whether you are eating due to hunger, habit, or your mood (e.g. due to sadness or anxiety).

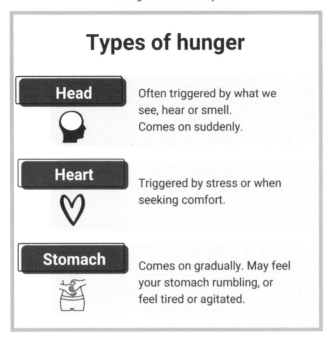

To get started you could try the following exercise below for 60 seconds during a meal.

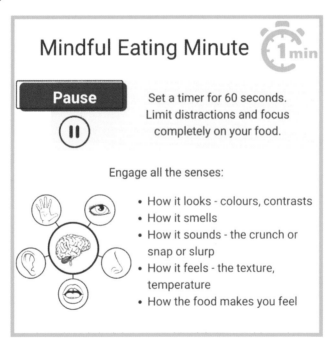

If you find you are comfort-eating, don't be too hard on yourself. It's useful to be aware of it and to then think of possible solutions you could try.

By eating mindfully, you will be better able to distinguish physical and emotional hunger and assess fullness and satisfaction much better.

Regular activity

Activity uses calories and increases our metabolic rate however weight management is not a simple calories in and calories out equation. How we sleep, how stressed we feel, how connected we are to appetite and the health of our microbiome all affect aspects of weight management.

Activity supports healthy weight management by helping to reduce stress, improving sleep quality, stimulating our body to build muscle and maintain bone (weight bearing activity), and may also have a positive effect on our microbiome.

Being active is so much more than weight management. Improved circulation supports good heart health which is more important post-menopause. It helps us to feel fitter and stronger, which can help us feel more confident with our bodies. Including activity into your day can also be a way to build social activity and prevent isolation.

Physical activity is an important part of managing menopause well. Making activity something that you enjoy is important. It can be something structured like a gym class or being part of a sports club. It can also be walking, dancing, yoga, gardening or cycling.

Diets and eating patterns

With the greater awareness and openness about menopause comes the plethora of diets and eating regimes that are sold as the perfect one for menopause such as 'Lose the menopause belly', eat for your hormones to control menopausal weight gain etc.

Many 'menopause diets' can result in limiting food groups and, as a consequence, limit the intake of nutrients important to aspects of menopausal and post-menopausal health. For example, eating too little protein can affect muscle strength and restricting carbohydrates may result in poorer gut health which is linked to heart health, mood and depression. As we go through the chapters we will highlight the importance of a range of nutrients on aspects of health and menopause.

Ultimately, food is not a simple case of calories, and health is not simply related to weight on the scales. In our Myths and Marketing chapter we touch upon a few diets that are often highlighted as being perfect for menopause.

The Mediterranean style of eating is the pattern of eating with the most evidence for supporting health through menopause and beyond. A recent analysis of UK data from 4,162 post-menopausal women suggests that following dietary guidelines, such as the UK's Eatwell Guide (PHE, 2018) or a Mediterranean diet, is associated with lower gains in waist circumference and a reduced risk of abdominal obesity in post-menopausal women. (Best & Flannery, 2023)

We will outline what the Mediterranean style of eating looks like in the Heart Health chapter and, as we go through the chapters, the benefits of it on many aspects of menopausal health will be explained.

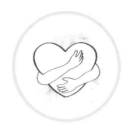

Heart Health

Underdiagnosed, understudied, undertreated and under recognised globally

Heart disease affects women too

A study in the Lancet in 2021 (Vogel et al., 2021) highlighted that not enough is being done to address the burden of heart disease in women. The conclusion of the report was that heart disease among women is underdiagnosed, treatment is poorer and the specific research on heart disease in women is lacking. This is despite the knowledge that there are differences in how heart disease presents itself between genders.

People may be surprised to be told that coronary heart disease kills more than twice as many women in the UK as breast cancer. (BHF, 2022) When we think of heart attacks, heart bypass surgery and stents we generally think of men. Heart disease is often thought of as a man's disease.

Much of the heart health advice given to the general population is based on research carried out in men and then applied to everyone, there is no nuance between gender. We need to be using research findings from studies in women to provide targeted information to improve women's cardiovascular health. This is particularly important as women approach menopause and beyond.

The Lancet report recommended that there be more done to raise awareness of cardiovascular disease in women. This chapter is dedicated to just that, with advice better tailored to women with current evidence available.

How menopause impacts women's heart health

Cholesterol levels

Raised cholesterol is one of the main risk factors for poor heart health. Oestrogen levels seem to be connected to blood cholesterol and as a result offers some protection against heart disease. We can see this by comparing blood cholesterol between men and women over time. There is a clear switch from men having higher cholesterol levels to women in those years around the average age of menopause. Data from the Health Survey for England in 2019 showed two in three women (66%) of women aged 55-64 years have raised cholesterol. (NHS Digital, 2020)

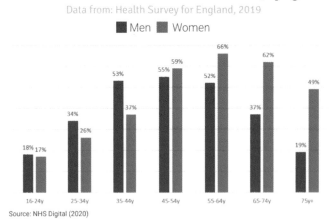

Proportion of adults with raised total cholesterol, by age and sex

Data from: Health Survey for England, 2019

Source: NHS Digital (2020)

The decrease in oestrogen during the menopause transition is associated with an increase in total cholesterol and low density lipoprotein (LDL) cholesterol, known as 'bad' cholesterol.

It is important to have an understanding of your cholesterol levels and have them checked regularly in those years approaching menopause and beyond. It can come as a surprise to be told that cholesterol levels are suddenly raised. There are however, many simple changes to your diet that can help to move back towards a healthier blood cholesterol profile.

Blood pressure

Blood pressure increases with age and this increase is steeper in post-menopausal women compared with men of similar age. Oestrogen helps relax and widen blood vessels so blood can flow more easily. This benefit is lost post-menopause. Menopausal symptoms, such as increased anxiety, poor sleep or reduced activity may also contribute to a rise in blood pressure.

There are plenty of dietary and lifestyle actions that we can take to help slow the increase in blood pressure.

Body fat storage

As we saw in the Healthy Weight Management chapter, the rate of weight gain increases during the menopausal transition and, more importantly, where body fat is stored changes. Post-menopausal women store more body fat around the middle and around organs including the heart. Weight carried around the middle, moving from a 'pear' to an 'apple' shape, is associated with a higher risk of heart disease and type 2 diabetes.

Keeping physically active and eating well can contribute to heart health especially if we keep our waist measurement to half our height. (NICE 2022)

Is your waist half your height?

Start by cutting a piece of string to
the length of your height.

Fold the string in half and
wrap it around your middle.

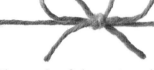

The ends of the string should
meet around your middle

If the two ends of the string struggle to meet you
are more at risk of heart disease and type 2 diabetes

The wider the gap, the bigger the health risk

Type 2 diabetes

Menopause may also impair how well your body controls blood sugar
adding to the risk of type 2 diabetes that we see due to the changes in
where fat is stored in the body. Type 2 diabetes risk can also increase
as we lose muscle mass, something that occurs naturally as we age.
(Slopien et al., 2018)

Type 2 diabetes and raised blood sugar levels can damage blood
vessels carrying blood to the heart and brain so affecting our heart and
circulatory health.

Introducing the Mediterranean style of eating

The Mediterranean Diet is often cited as being the best style of eating
for a healthy heart and overall wellness. We will be referring to this style
of eating regularly throughout the book. Not only is it considered to be
one of the best patterns of eating for heart health, there are lots of

reasons why it is also very helpful in maintaining good health during and beyond the menopause.

It is thought to help support a healthy gut microbiome, which we talk about in more detail later. This may be the reason why this pattern of eating may be so beneficial on risk factors for heart disease, such as reducing blood cholesterol levels and supporting the immune response.

The Mediterranean style of eating focuses on plant-based eating including a diverse range of plant foods such as wholegrains, legumes, fruits and vegetables, with moderate amounts of fish, dairy, eggs and poultry. Red meat is eaten occasionally and sweet foods are consumed but fruit is the preferred dessert. Alcohol is consumed but in moderation and usually with food. This style of eating encourages the use of oils rich in unsaturated fats (mono- and poly-unsaturated fats) like olive or rapeseed (canola) oil, as well as nuts and seeds.

A great deal of research has been carried out on the Mediterranean way of eating that originated in the coastal regions of the Mediterranean. This pattern of eating is also reflected in other areas of the world with long life and good heart health with different ingredients, the Nordic diet and the traditional Japanese way of eating are just two examples.

How a Mediterranean diet helps heart health

More heart healthy fats

There are a greater variety of fats in this way of eating and this leads to a lower amount of saturated fats. There are higher amounts of unsaturated fats that are found in fish, seeds and other plant sources.

There are less saturated fats from fatty meats, butter, ghee, palm and coconut oils, and the products made using these (i.e. pastries, fried foods, cakes and biscuits). Instead more heart healthy unsaturated fats from olive oil or rapeseed oil, vegetable spreads, nuts and seeds are used.

This supports better cholesterol management and healthy blood vessels.

Fish is a regular feature in this way of eating. Oil-rich fish are a great source of healthy unsaturated fats, particularly omega-3 which help maintain normal cholesterol levels and normal heart function. Including one or two portions of oily fish per week, such as salmon, trout, sardines or mackerel is recommended.

Including a range of plant sources of omega-3, such as rapeseed oil, walnuts, chia seeds, hemp seeds and flaxseeds, helps achieve a good mix of fats.

 Oily fish are one of the few foods that contain vitamin D. As well as being beneficial for bone health, vitamin D may have a role in heart health too.

Wholegrains and other fibre-rich foods

The focus of plant foods includes wholegrains which often don't get a lot of attention. Wholegrains provide a variety of B-vitamins and some minerals such as magnesium, iron and zinc that are beneficial for heart health. Including more wholegrain foods in the diet has been shown to reduce risk of cardiovascular disease. (Reynolds et al., 2019)

Wholegrain foods include wholemeal bread and cereals, brown rice, rye, buckwheat, quinoa, oats and barley. Including at least three servings of wholegrain foods every day is thought to provide the greatest benefit. (Aune et al., 2016)

The fibre contained in wholegrains is also important for heart health. Including lots of plant food means fibre-rich foods such as beans, peas, vegetables, fruits, nuts and seeds. The more variety you can include in your diet, the better.

In the UK, we currently eat much less than the recommended 30g fibre a day. (Public Health England, 2016) Add more plant foods to increase fibre gradually, making sure you keep well hydrated to avoid gut issues like bloating.

Oats and barley contain a particular type of soluble fibre called beta-glucan, which can help lower cholesterol if you have 3g or more of it daily, as part of a healthy diet. Including porridge or overnight oats, oat-based breakfast cereal, oatcakes, adding oat bran to soups or smoothies or adding pearl barley to stews or a salad are useful options.

More plant proteins and less red and processed meat

Meat and other animal foods are not the sole focus for protein sources. Many plants that provide good amounts of protein feature. Including foods such as lentils, beans, peas, Quorn™, soya mince, tofu, nuts and seeds help to reduce the quantity of animal foods. As well as providing protein, they are naturally lower in saturated fat whilst providing heart healthy unsaturated fats and fibre. In addition, they give this style of eating a more rounded nutrition profile compared to those that are heavier on animal proteins.

There is lots of evidence that soya foods such as tofu, soya mince, edamame beans and soya alternatives to milk and yoghurt, are beneficial for heart health as they help lower cholesterol levels and blood pressure. (Ramdath et al., 2017, Kou et al., 2017)

Soya foods tend to be naturally rich in high quality protein and low in saturated fat as well as providing fibre, vitamins, minerals and soya isoflavones (a type of plant oestrogen) that are beneficial for heart health. Including two servings soya foods daily can benefit heart health and may help manage menopausal hot flushes. (see Hot Flushes chapter)

Include at least 5-a-day

Mediterranean style eating is rich in fruits and vegetables with fruit being commonly consumed as dessert and sweet snacks. We know, from many studies, that including at least five portions (400g) of fruit and vegetables a day is associated with a reduced risk of cardiovascular disease. (Aune et al., 2017) In the Mediterranean region, local fresh fruits and vegetables are a huge part of the food culture, however we can't always have farm fresh local produce. It is important to remember that it really doesn't have to be fresh and local. Fresh, frozen, canned or dried fruit and vegetables all count. Whatever is affordable and available for you is fine.

Fruits and vegetables, in addition to the fibre they add to the diet, contain a variety of heart healthy nutrients such as vitamin C, carotenoids, potassium and antioxidants. These all promote a healthy vascular system.

Adding more fruit and vegetables to your meals and snacks can help reduce or replace foods that we would prefer to eat less of like those high in saturated fat, sugar and salt.

Cut down on salt

In the Mediterranean, there is a big focus on using local herbs, lemon juice and other flavours. Being inspired to use other flavours like citrus, vinegar, spices, herbs and black pepper can help to reduce the need for salt. This is important to reduce blood pressure.

The focus on food and cooking with minimally processed and local produce results in less consumption of processed foods. As 75% of our salt intake is already in the foods we buy, such as bread, savoury snacks, sauces and ready meals (NHS, 2021), this approach can be helpful.

We can't always cook from scratch, however there are lots of ways of using convenience products or store cupboard items that lower our salt intake. It's worth checking product labels for the salt content and opt for those lower in salt. Aim to keep your salt intakes below 6g a day .

 Use the free 'Food Switch' app to scan a product barcode and to see how much salt is in the product and what similar but healthier alternative products there are. (Action on Salt, 2022)

A portion of nuts a day

Nuts are a commonly used in cooking and for snacks. Nuts contain cholesterol-lowering fats and fibre as well as vitamins and minerals that benefit heart health. Nuts have a relatively high energy content, but evidence shows that including a daily portion of nuts (30g, or roughly a closed handful) helps reduce total cholesterol and LDL cholesterol (also known a 'bad' cholesterol), and is not associated with weight gain. (Kim et al., 2018)

Foods with added plant stanols and sterols

Plant stanols and sterols are naturally present in plant foods such as vegetable oils, seeds, grains and legumes – all of which feature in the Mediterranean diet. These compounds have a similar chemical structure to cholesterol so they partially block some cholesterol absorption which has the effect of lowering the amount of cholesterol in the blood.

If you have raised cholesterol, the amount found in plant foods is not enough to have an effect, however, an intake of 1.5g-3g of plant stanols and sterols per day is recommended to reduce cholesterol. (Heart UK, 2022) For those who do not have high blood cholesterol levels there is no real benefit taking these products.

There are a wide range of food products now available with added sterols and stanols. Look out for mini drinks, yoghurts, milk and spreads fortified with stanols and sterols. The manufacturers of these products have lots of information on their websites on how to include them to maximise the benefit.

Other aspects of lifestyle

In areas where this style of eating is prominent, and where people live long and healthier lives, they tend to share some other non-diet lifestyle factors that also promote good heart health.

Physical activity is part of daily life and they have strong communities with lower levels of stress. It seems that the Mediterranean diet is about more than just the food.

- Walking every day or using a bike as your main means of transport can be very positive for heart health, in addition to more formal exercise that you might do.

- Breaking up long periods spent sitting, with walking or standing, can help make your blood and circulatory system more efficient and help keep your blood pressure down.

- A good night's sleep and other things that help reduce stress are very positive as stress hormones raise our blood pressure and may increase inflammation.

- Smoking can narrow your arteries and make your blood more likely to clot. If you do smoke, seek help to stop. There's information on the NHS website on support services. (NHS, 2022)

- Limit alcohol intake to no more than 2-3 units per day and consume no more than 14 units of alcohol per week, with some alcohol-free days in between.

- Have a social network or connect with friends and family regularly.

Not only do these promote good heart health, all of these things help to support the management of menopausal symptoms.

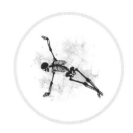

Bone Health

How does menopause affect my bones?
Am I at risk of osteoporosis?

Bone health through life

When we are born, if we were to have an x-ray we would not be able to see all of the skeleton. The cartilage has yet to be mineralised and so it is invisible to x-ray. The skeleton not only grows as we do but it becomes denser through mineralisation. We can measure this density, or our bone mass. Once we stop growing, our skeleton continues to develop and increase its strength, with our bone mass continuing to increase, peaking at around 30 years. Our optimal peak bone mass is determined by our genes. Whether we can achieve it is dependent on our lifestyle and diet.

After this, our bones start to become less dense very slowly in both men and women. Oestrogen slows this loss of bone, as it is involved in bone turnover. As a result, women have a steeper loss of bone during menopause. This makes women at a much greater risk of osteoporosis than men. Half of all women over the age of 50 will suffer a fracture due to poor bone health compared to 20% of men. (Royal Osteoporosis Society, 2020)

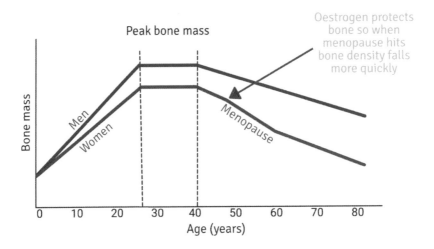

Osteoporosis occurs when bone loss reaches a certain point causing a loss of integrity to the fine honeycomb structure which gives bones their lightweight strength. The structure becomes open and airy losing density and strength. The bones become brittle and fragile. Fractures happen easily and can result in loss of independence, pain and ill-health. The vertebrae in the spine can crumble resulting in back pain and deformity.

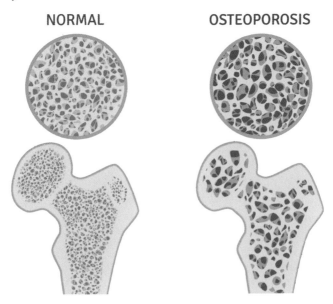

Am I at risk of osteoporosis?

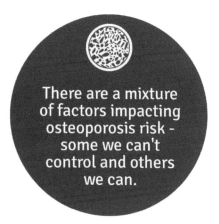

There are a mixture of factors impacting osteoporosis risk - some we can't control and others we can.

Osteoporosis often runs in families. If osteoporosis is something that has affected your female relatives, you may be at higher risk. Early menopause increases your risk of osteoporosis as can drug treatments such as long term steroid treatment or certain cancer drugs.

Bones respond to the weight they carry. People who are lighter and very slender tend to be more at risk than people who are of a heavier build. Low body weight (a BMI of under 19) is also thought to increase risk of osteoporosis, partly due to less weight but also body fat stores help to maintain oestrogen levels. (BDA, 2019)

Weight bearing and muscle strengthening activity such as brisk walking, jogging, resistance training or dancing helps stimulate bone formation and is hugely important for building and maintaining strong bones. Inactivity can increase your risk.

We know that diet is important to the health of our bones. Bone is made up of protein fibres which are strengthened with minerals such as calcium. Vitamin D is essential for calcium to be incorporated into our bones. If we look at the National Diet and Nutrition Survey in the UK, nearly 1 in 6 adults have low levels of vitamin D. (Public Health England, 2020)

Vegan diets have become much more common in recent years and a study has shown that vegans had a 43% higher risk of bone fractures than meat eaters. The authors of the study, looking at data from almost 55,000 men and women in the UK, state that this might be due to a combination of lower average body mass index (BMI), and lower average intakes of calcium and protein in vegans. (Tong et al, 2020)

Evidence shows that smoking increases the risk of osteoporosis, as does drinking a lot of alcohol. There is no need to go tee-total, as evidence shows that a moderate amount of alcohol may be protective. If you do drink alcohol, staying within government guidelines is advised. To read more about the guidelines and ways to cut down on alcohol see the Drink Less website on our Links and Resources page.

All of these factors are considered along with measurements of bone mineral density to consider your risk of fracture. The Royal Osteoporosis Society is a fantastic source of information via their website and social media streams.

Tips to protect bone health after menopause

There is nothing we can do about our genes and we can't go back and change anything about our younger lives. However there is a lot you can do now to protect your bones and reduce your risk of osteoporosis. Here are a few tips:

Calcium - eat plenty of calcium-rich foods

Milk and dairy products are the richest sources of calcium and make a big contribution to our calcium intakes – figures show that 34–44% of the calcium intake in adults comes from dairy, depending on age. (Public Health England, 2020) In addition to dairy foods like yoghurt, cheese and milk, the following foods can contribute calcium to your diet:

- If you use dairy alternatives, always choose brands that are fortified with calcium and vitamin D.
- Choose soya products, such as soya alternatives to yoghurt fortified with calcium, firm tofu which has been set with calcium (check the ingredients label for calcium sulphate or calcium chloride), edamame beans and soya and linseed bread.

- Canned fish with edible bones like sardines and mackerel are a brilliant source of calcium.

- Wholemeal, brown or white bread (in the UK calcium is added to all white and brown bread).

- Green vegetables, such as broccoli, kale and Pak choi.

- Sesame seeds (or sesame tahini), almonds, chia seeds and sunflower seeds.

 Shake the carton of fortified non-dairy milk alternatives. Added calcium can sink to the bottom to be thrown away with the carton. (Heaney & Rafferty, 2006)

Women often ask whether there is any need to take a calcium supplement, however, if you eat plenty of calcium-rich foods it is unlikely that you need to. Taking high intakes of calcium above what you need can increase your risk of kidney stones and high levels of calcium in the blood can make you unwell.

Calcium can bind to certain compounds in some plant foods such as the phytates and oxalates in some green leafy vegetables. By eating a range of different foods across the day you reduce the effect of these interactions. Foods that may bind with minerals like calcium are foods that contain lots of important nutrients so shouldn't be avoided.

If you have an underactive thyroid, calcium and thyroid medication compete for the same transfer sites in the gut so it is best to take your medication away from meals rich in calcium as your dose of thyroxine may not be achieved in reality.

Vitamin D - take a supplement, eat some oily fish and get outdoors

Not only does vitamin D allow our bones to incorporate calcium, it also helps our gut absorb calcium from our food. We can increase our vitamin D in the following ways:

- Take a vitamin D supplement of 10 micrograms (µg) or 400 IU (International Units) per day, preferably with a meal. Vitamin D is fat-soluble and fat in the meal helps absorption.

- Eat foods that contribute to vitamin D:

  - Oily fish (such as: mackerel, salmon, trout, sardines, herring, anchovies)
  - Eggs
  - Fortified foods, such as some non-dairy alternatives to milk and yoghurt and breakfast cereals
  - Vitamin D enhanced mushrooms

- In northern latitudes like the UK, between March and October, get outside in the sunshine without sunscreen for 10 minute bursts once or twice a day when your shadow is shorter than your height. If you have darker skin, it takes longer to produce vitamin D. Do not let your skin burn.

 Did you know that if you leave regular mushrooms on a sunny windowsill for an hour or so, it increases their vitamin D content? (Cardwell et al. 2018)

Protein - spaced throughout the day

When we think of protein we think of our muscles. However, protein is also extremely important for the maintenance of healthy bones. Protein forms a mesh within bones which is strengthened by minerals attaching to it. Without sufficient protein we cannot maintain the strength of our bones.

Eating sufficient protein throughout the day also maintains our muscles which allows us to keep active, supporting the health of our bones. As we age we also begin to gradually lose muscle, which affects our strength and weight, which, in turn, affects our bone strength. It is also true that our protein requirements increase slightly as we get older, even though energy requirements fall and appetite can get smaller for many people.

Sports nutrition tells us protein is used by the body more efficiently if intake is spread out across the day and when we consume protein after physical activity. It's useful to include some protein foods at every meal. Meat, fish, eggs, and dairy (for example milk, cheese and yoghurt) provide high quality protein. Good plant sources of protein include soya products (such as soya alternatives to milk and yoghurt and tofu), cereals, beans, peas, lentils, nuts and seeds.

Diets in the UK generally provide adequate protein but our protein intake may not be spread well across the day. An easy way to improve the spread across the day is to add protein to breakfast with food such as nuts and seeds, a soya yoghurt alternative or eggs. We've made some suggestions within our recipes for adding protein.

Collagen

Collagen gets spoken about a lot in relation to menopause. Collagen is important for connective tissue and this includes our bones, joints and our skin. As we age, our collagen production falls.

Collagen production requires protein, and more specifically a range of amino acids that provide the building blocks for protein. A diet containing a wide range of protein foods consumed throughout the day can provide the protein and amino acids needed. You do not have to eat foods that are rich in pre-made collagen like bone broth, chicken skin, dishes made from cheaper cuts of meat high in connective tissue that are cooked long and slow, fish skin etc. Focus on including a wide range of protein foods across the day such as fish, eggs, dairy foods, soya foods, meat and nuts and seeds.

In addition to amino acids, the body needs a range of micronutrients found in plant foods to allow these amino acids to be converted into collagen, the most famous being vitamin C. Severe vitamin C deficiency is the cause of scurvy which is visible by the body's connective tissue essentially falling apart.

A Mediterranean style diet will provide the nutrients necessary for collagen production. Smoking and too much alcohol interfere with collagen production. This may be why these are both associated with increased risk of osteoporosis.

We discuss collagen supplements in the Myths and Marketing chapter.

Physical activity

Activity is good for many of the effects of menopause. For activity to benefit our bones, it needs to be weight-bearing as this stimulates the process of reinforcing the protein mesh and its mineralisation. Walking, climbing stairs, jogging, gardening, dancing and exercise classes are all good examples of weight-bearing activity.

If you do any physical activity, having a protein containing snack afterwards is a good way to help your body to use protein most efficiently. Our muscles are most able to use protein in the hour or so directly after exercise.

Simple protein containing snacks include hummus, nut butter on toast or in a smoothie, oatcakes with a little cheese or a milky drink.

Speak to your doctor

If you think that you are at high risk, maybe because you have female relatives who have osteoporosis or you have experienced an early menopause, talk to your doctor. Bone density can be measured and your specific risk factors assessed. You may be offered hormone replacement therapy as this can help to reduce bone loss and there is medication available that can be used if your risk is high.

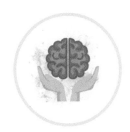

Mood and Mental Health

Can diet lessen the effects that menopause has on emotions and mood?

Menopause and mental health

Many women navigating menopause report symptoms such as mood swings, anxiety, insomnia and difficulties with memory and concentration. The drop in oestrogen affects the brain directly and through interactions with neurotransmitters that influence our emotions, anxiety, sleep and mood. In particular, oestrogen is connected to the production and potency of serotonin, which is linked to sleep, mood and executive function. Many women ask about the extent diet can play a role to alleviate these effects.

Diet and neurotransmitters

Neurotransmitters are essential for our brain to function and communicate with our body. They are essential for us to feel things like hunger, joy and anxiety but also to process tasks in our brain like keeping track of several things, and remembering where we put our keys whilst being distracted by the phone ringing. If we can optimise our body's ability to produce neurotransmitters through what we eat, we may limit the effect of the drop in hormones on their potency.

Protein is necessary for the production of serotonin and other neurotransmitters important to mood and brain function, specific amino acids are needed to build their structure. Protein is made up of chains of amino acids. It is individual amino acids that our bodies require to build our own proteins - our hormones and neurotransmitters are proteins. Some amino acids we can make ourselves but there are some that are essential from our diet. Neurotransmitters require essential amino acids for their production.

Some neurotransmitters are made in the gut by the microbes living there. The most well-known of these is serotonin. Ninety percent of this neurotransmitter is made in our gut. It is therefore, really important to look after our gut health to optimise the production of neurotransmitters.

Focus on serotonin

Serotonin is often dubbed the happiness hormone and oestrogen has an effect on potency and production of this neurotransmitter. It is also important in aspects of executive function – working memory and concentration for example. Menopausal 'brain fog' may be, in part related to the effect that a drop in oestrogen has on serotonin. It is important to note that while this may feel like dementia kicking in, it is not a sign of cognitive decline.

To make serotonin we need a particular amino acid called tryptophan. Foods that are good sources of tryptophan include chicken, beef, pork, fish, seafood, tofu, soybeans, seeds, oats, bananas, eggs, milk and other dairy products.

Consuming foods containing tryptophan may help to compensate for the loss of the serotonin enhancing effect of oestrogen by maximising the production of this important neurotransmitter.

Other neurotransmitters and amino acids

Other neurotransmitters involved in our moods and emotions include dopamine, GABA and norepinephrine. By optimising their production we may have a positive effect on the emotional aspects of menopause. There is less evidence of there being a direct connection with oestrogen. GABA (gamma-acetyl butyric acid) has an important role in reducing anxiety.

Essential amino acids vital for production of these neurotransmitters are tyrosine, phenylethylalanine and glutamine. Most of the foods which contain tryptophan also contain one or other of these amino acids. In addition to the foods containing tryptophan, we can also include other foods containing one or more of these three essential amino acids such as wholegrains, beans, nuts, leafy vegetables and avocado.

Carbohydrate link

Foods rich in carbohydrates can help to boost the uptake and use of tryptophan by clearing the amino acids that get in the way of our body using tryptophan. When we eat carbohydrate rich foods, insulin in our blood clears these amino acids from our blood stream along with sugar, leaving tryptophan more available to us.

In addition, foods providing good quality carbohydrate are extremely important for the bacteria living in our gut. By feeding our microbiome we support the gut's role in producing and releasing the neurotransmitters that are so important to our mental health.

The gut and mental health connection

We are seeing more evidence that if we nourish our gut bacteria with the right diet, we can improve our mental health. The main nerve connecting the brain and the gut is called the vagus nerve. This enables a two-way communication channel. The neurotransmitters produced by the gut and its microbiome can communicate with the body independently of the vagus nerve, for example travelling through the bloodstream. They also produce chemicals that regulate hunger and satiety.

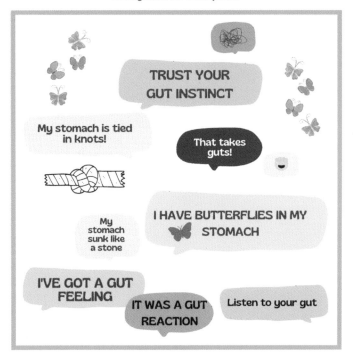

The main way to keep our gut microbiome happy is to feed it well by including a diverse range of carbohydrates and fibre - choosing higher fibre foods where possible. Plant foods are key, and as wide a variety as possible including: fruits, vegetables, wholegrains, beans, legumes, nuts and seeds, as well as herbs and spices.

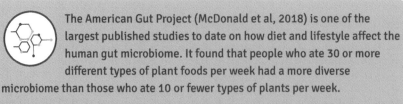

The American Gut Project (McDonald et al, 2018) is one of the largest published studies to date on how diet and lifestyle affect the human gut microbiome. It found that people who ate 30 or more different types of plant foods per week had a more diverse microbiome than those who ate 10 or fewer types of plants per week.

This diversity seems to be key to health. Having more diverse plant foods in the diet supports a diverse and well-functioning microbiome that results in the most health benefits.

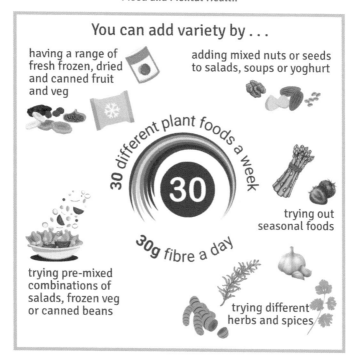

We can also contribute to our gut health by consuming fermented foods, such as live yoghurt, kefir, kombucha and sourdough bread. Ways that fermented foods might help to diversify and feed our gut include:

1. 'Live' products (such as yoghurt and kefir) contain beneficial bacteria or 'probiotics', which may pass through to our gut to add to our microbiome.

2. The fermentation process breaks down food components that feed our microbiome directly - food for our microbiome is referred to as 'prebiotics'.

Foods that have certain types of fibre or other compounds that feed our microbiome, either naturally or as an extra ingredient, are also referred to as 'prebiotics'.

The Mediterranean diet and mood

A Mediterranean style of eating, as we have seen already, is a diet rich in plant foods and is considered a way of eating that supports gut health. It has been the focus of the effect of diet on mood and mental health. There are other aspects of this way of eating that may support mood in addition to its positive effect on the gut microbiome.

Studies have shown that eating a Mediterranean diet may reduce the risk of depression. (Shaffiei et al., 2019; Jacka et al., 2017) This is likely to be due to a combination of elements of this diet. Including plenty of fibre-rich plant foods supportive of gut health also provides a range of vitamins, minerals and antioxidants thought to benefit the brain and mood. Oily fish, a key element of this diet is the best dietary source of long-chain omega-3 fatty acids known as EPA (eicosapentaenoic acid) and DHA (docosahexaenoic acid). These are particularly beneficial for brain function.

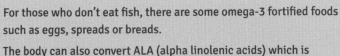

For those who don't eat fish, there are some omega-3 fortified foods such as eggs, spreads or breads.

The body can also convert ALA (alpha linolenic acids) which is another omega-3 found in plant foods, such as hemp, chia and pumpkin seeds, walnuts and rapeseed oil, into EPA and DHA. However, the conversion process is not very efficient as less than 15% of ALA is converted into EPA or DHA. (NIH, 2022)

An omega-3 supplement containing EPA and DHA can be beneficial for vegetarians, vegans and those who don't eat any oily fish.

The Mediterranean diet provides a variety of B-vitamins which are needed for releasing energy from the food we eat. Low levels of B-vitamins can lead to feeling tired, depressed or irritable. Meat, fish, eggs and dairy as well as wholegrains, fortified cereals, soya beans, nuts and some fruits and vegetables provide B-vitamins.

Vitamin B12 is found in almost all foods of animal origin. If you don't eat meat, fish, eggs or dairy foods, then a vitamin B12 supplement is recommended. Including plant foods fortified with vitamin B12 is also useful for those following a vegan or mainly plant-based diet.

Other factors that may benefit mental health

Eat regular meals and snacks

The brain relies on a steady supply of energy (in the form of glucose), ideally from foods such as wholegrains, beans, nuts, seeds, fruits and vegetables that are digested slowly to provide a steady supply of glucose to the brain. Diets with lots of refined carbohydrates and sugars will result in quick bursts of energy, followed by big dips leading to low energy, poor concentration and cravings for more sugary foods. Eating regular meals and snacks can help the body balance blood sugar levels. Mindful eating can be a useful practice to help us recognise our feelings of physical hunger so that we can respond to them by having a meal or a snack to help level out the peaks and dips in energy.

Keeping well hydrated

Keeping well hydrated is important as evidence shows that even slight dehydration may affect brain function and mood. Aim to drink 1.5 to 2 litres of fluid a day. Avoiding too much caffeine from coffee and fizzy drinks is useful as too much, particularly if you are sensitive to it, may result in irritability and headache.

Limit alcohol

Having an alcoholic drink may result in feeling more relaxed and less anxious, but these effects wear off quickly. Alcohol is a depressant, which can disrupt the balance of neurotransmitters in the brain. This can impact our mood, sleep and menopause symptoms. Stay within the recommended 14 units of alcohol per week or, if you're experiencing anxiety or low mood, cutting it out completely may be the best option. See the Hot Flushes chapter for the low risk drinking guidelines.

Regular physical activity and movement

Physical activity has numerous benefits for both physical and mental health. When we are physically active our body releases hormones in our brain that contribute to reduced stress, improved mood, improved brain function and better sleep quality. Regular physical activity among peri-menopausal women helps reduce depression, anxiety and improves satisfaction with life. Even relatively brief moderate-intensity activity such as walking seems to trigger a reduction in depressive symptoms. (Hybholt, 2022) Activities such as yoga and dancing have also been found to have a positive effect on self-esteem of peri-menopausal women. (Hybholt, 2022)

Adequate sleep

Disruption of sleep is a common menopause symptom. Not getting adequate sleep can have a negative impact on our health and well-being. The drop in oestrogen can lead to mood changes and poor sleep can further exacerbate this. The decline of oestrogen, testosterone and progesterone can lead to anxiety, restlessness and disrupted sleep. It can be a challenging time for women, and we hope the chapter on Sleeping Well will be helpful.

Feeling connected

Isolation can impact our mental health. Simply spending some time with like-minded people, friends that lift you and doing things that you enjoy is invaluable for maintaining good mental health and managing stress.

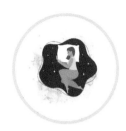

Sleeping Well

Does menopause affect sleep and can my diet improve it?

Menopause and sleep

Sleep is so important to health and is something that is impacted by menopause. Between 28 and 63% of women experience sleep disturbance during the menopause. (WHC, 2021) From a cohort of 25,570 peri-menopausal females from the smartphone-based ZOE Health App, the most commonly reported menopausal symptoms included sleep problems (68% of women), night sweats (60%), mood changes (60%) and hot flashes (59%). (Bermingham K and Berry, S personal communication, Apr 11, 2023)

The effect of menopause on sleep is a mixture of direct effects of hormones, the impact of menopausal symptoms and the effect of age on sleep. Lack of sleep can in turn exacerbate menopausal symptoms and negatively affect post-menopausal health.

The changes in hormone levels during menopause can have effects that impact sleep. Oestrogen has been shown to reduce the time it takes to fall asleep, reduce the number of awakenings during sleep and increases total sleep time. Oestrogen also has a role in regulating body temperature and helps keep the core body temperature low during the night. (Lee et al., 2019) Hormone replacement therapy has been shown to improve sleep quality in menopausal women. (Pan et al., 2022)

Common symptoms of menopause are definite enemies of good sleep. Many women report that hot flushes and night sweats interrupt sleep significantly. Lesser known 'restless legs syndrome' (see below), can also result in significant sleep disturbances. In addition, peri-menopausal women often report more frequent night time toilet trips also interfering with a good night's sleep. We explore the relationship between oestrogen and bladder function in the Healthy Hydration chapter.

Menopausal women can be more prone to anxiety which can make sleep harder and a lack of sleep can aggravate mood and anxiety, therefore, there can be a self-fulfilling cycle. Read more in the Mood and Mental Health chapter.

Melatonin, which is a hormone involved in the sleep-wake cycle, falls with age. As the drop in oestrogen impacts melatonin, the effect on normal sleeping patterns is greater in women than in older men. Menopause is associated with a significant reduction of melatonin levels. (Jehan et al., 2015)

melatonin

[mel-uh-toh-nin]

n.) A natural hormone produced in the pineal gland in the brain. It's production is responsive to light, levels increase at night and fall during the day. It helps regulate the sleep-wake cycle.

Restless Legs Syndrome

Restless Legs Syndrome is very simply characterised by an overwhelming urge to move the legs. Movement provides a temporary relief from the unpleasant crawling or creeping sensation felt in the legs (or other parts of the body). First described in 1672, why it occurs is still not very clear and despite its negative impact, the syndrome is often under-diagnosed and inadequately treated. (Harrison et al., 2019)

Although it can occur at any time of day, it is most often felt during the evening or overnight, which leads to disrupted sleep. For those most badly affected, it can lead to significant insomnia that affects health. Restless Legs Syndrome is almost twice as common in women as it is in men. One study found 15% of women aged 18-64 years experienced these symptoms (Wesstrom et al., 2008) and it is more common in women going through menopause.

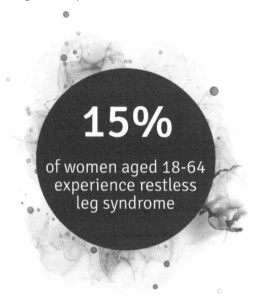

15%

of women aged 18-64 experience restless leg syndrome

As iron and magnesium levels seem to dip at night and as Restless Legs Syndrome seems to be more common at night, it is thought that these nutrients may be important. Vitamin D may be linked with Restless Legs Syndrome. However, not enough studies have been carried out to get a clear understanding of how diet might affect this uncomfortable syndrome.

It may be helpful to keep active during the day, avoid sitting for long periods and doing some gentle exercise or stretching in the evening. A 12-week study found that 30 minutes of daily yoga decreased symptoms in adults with Restless Legs Syndrome. (Innes et al., 2020)

Avoiding smoking and drinking alcohol and having a regular bedtime routine may also help manage the symptoms. There are some treatment options available, so talk to your GP for advice, especially if it is causing you trouble sleeping.

The toilet calls in the night

Sleep can also be disrupted by waking in the night to empty the bladder. Having to get up more than twice a night is considered to affect health by the very fact that it reduces sleep. It has a name – nocturia.

Nocturia gets more common as we get older, in both men and women. It is thought that the weakening circadian rhythm in older adults is responsible. Melatonin is not the only hormone that increases as it gets dark. Hormones are released to suppress the kidneys to slow the filling of the bladder during the night to allow a more sound sleep. A weaker sleep-wake cycle means this doesn't happen which results in waking up to empty the bladder.

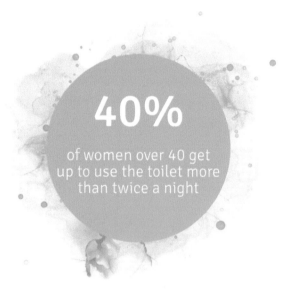

40%
of women over 40 get up to use the toilet more than twice a night

Women are affected much more than men, with some figures suggesting that around 40% of women over 40 report nocturia. (Leslie et al., 2022) The fact that melatonin drops more significantly in women around menopause may explain some of the difference. However we know that oestrogen directly affects the pelvic region in ways that impacts bladder function and risk of urinary tract infections.

One way to reduce nocturia is to taper your fluid intake in the hours before bedtime – this has been proven to help. Many women do this either subconsciously or actively. It is really important that this does not lead to an overall drop in daily fluid intake – the reduction later in the day needs to be accounted for earlier in the day or you risk becoming dehydrated. See more in the Healthy Hydration chapter.

We know that topical vaginal oestrogen can reduce nocturia in menopausal women (Akhavizadegan et al., 2018) and that other issues relating to feelings of increased frequency and urgency can often be treated in other ways. It is important to talk to your GP if your bladder function is beginning to be noticeably more inconvenient or troublesome.

Sleep and health

Whilst an occasional poor night's sleep is unlikely to have much of an impact on your health, regular disrupted sleep can seriously affect your health and well-being, and in particular impact your risk of obesity, heart disease and diabetes.

Lack of sleep raises the level of stress hormones. This can have a negative effect on blood pressure and heart health. The gut is negatively affected, potentially worsening gut issues and impacting the health of the microbiome. It can have a negative effect on our appetite, making us more drawn to calorie-rich food and drink. This, in turn, can affect weight management.

Lack of sleep can also make us more emotional and affect our concentration and focus. The drop in oestrogen during menopause affects both our mood and executive function. Poor sleep exacerbates these effects.

It's agreed that lack of sleep is not good for us. However, do not despair. There are positive and practical things we can do to improve the quality of our sleep.

Diet and sleep

The neurotransmitter serotonin, often dubbed the 'happiness hormone', is key to good sleep. It has an important role in the production of melatonin, which controls our sleep-wake cycle. It is also important in mood and anxiety, which in turn play a role in sleep. If we are anxious or worried it is much harder to sleep well.

Our diet is important in the production of neurotransmitters, such as serotonin. Nutrients linked to better sleep seem to do this through their effect on our production of neurotransmitters.

Oestrogen and serotonin are known to interact. Diet is important in the production of serotonin, and by improving our diet, to support the production of neurotransmitters, we may dampen the effects of the drop in oestrogen.

Eating a plant-rich diet such as the Mediterranean diet has been associated with better sleep. (Scoditti et al., 2022) This type of diet provides natural food sources of tryptophan needed for serotonin production in order to make melatonin and also several foods that contain melatonin naturally, such as cherries, nuts and milk. (Meng et al., 2017)

Nutrients that may help with sleep

Magnesium

Magnesium is a nutrient that is often spoken of as important for sleep. It is important for the function of your nervous system. In relation to sleep more specifically, it is involved in making serotonin and regulating the hormone melatonin. This connection between magnesium and the hormone that helps control the sleep-wake cycle has led to a body of research exploring the magnesium sleep relationship. A review of 27 studies, (Ji et al., 2017) reported adequate magnesium was positively associated with how long people slept.

There are many sources of magnesium. Foods to look for include: fish, meat and dairy products, pumpkin seeds, wholemeal bread, spinach, peas, edamame beans, lentils, quinoa, Brazil nuts, almonds and flaxseeds.

Tryptophan

Tryptophan is an essential amino acid, one the body must obtain from the diet, that is an important building block for serotonin and melatonin. Foods rich in tryptophan include: poultry, eggs, cheese, fish, tofu and soya foods, milk, peanuts, pumpkin seeds and oily fish.

Vitamin B6, Calcium and Zinc

These three nutrients are all involved in the production and regulation of melatonin. Food sources of these nutrients include:

Vitamin B6 - poultry, pulses, lentils, bananas and soya foods

Calcium - dairy foods, tofu, fortified plant drinks and yoghurts

Zinc - meat, shellfish, cheese, bread, quinoa, pumpkin and sesame seeds

Vitamin D

When we think of vitamin D we often first think of bone health but there is evidence that it may also have a role to play in how well we sleep.

A review published in 2018 of nine studies, found that people with low vitamin D levels are more likely to sleep less and not as well. (Gao et al., 2018) A study has also shown that taking a vitamin D supplement can improve sleep quality in those with sleep disorders. (Majid et al., 2018)

The Government advice in the UK is that adults should take a vitamin D supplement of 10 μg (micrograms) a day. This is equivalent to 400 IU (International Units). See the Bone Health chapter to learn more about vitamin D.

Fibre and other compounds that improve gut health

Our gut is where the majority of our serotonin is produced. Poor gut health, which is a gut microbiome lacking in diversity of microbes or being unbalanced in some way, is associated with anxiety and stress which may lead to poorer sleep.

The best way to support our gut health is to include lots of variety in our diet, especially plant foods. These foods provide our gut microbes with fibres to feed on and keep our gut healthy.

We know that the gut microbiome is important for many aspects of our health. This may be in part due to its link to our brain. It works in the other direction too - poor sleep can disrupt the gut microbiome.

Read more about good gut health in the Mood and Mental Health chapter.

Foods and drinks that may help you sleep better

Drinks

Herbal teas with chamomile or valerian root are often chosen as caffeine free alternative hot drinks for later in the day. If you are not a fan of herbal tea but are a tea drinker then switching to a non-caffeinated version or a tea such as Rooibos can also be a good swap.

Drinking a warm malted milky drink may also help some people have a less restless sleep. There is something comforting about a milky drink before bed. Milk contains calcium, tryptophan and naturally occurring melatonin. The lactose and added sugars make the milk's tryptophan content more readily available for conversion to serotonin and melatonin production for better sleep. Maybe it is not so surprising that warm, milky drinks are such a bed time favourite.

Foods

Whilst it is beneficial to have a bit of gap between a big meal and bed time, going to bed feeling a little hungry may make it hard to sleep or cause you to wake up later. A light snack containing some of the nutrients important for melatonin production may help you sleep better. Here are a few suggestions:

- A small pot of yoghurt or soya yoghurt alternative with pumpkin seeds
- A few oatcakes with almond butter
- A small milk and banana smoothie
- A few crackers and cheese
- Dry roasted edamame beans with dried fruit

Things that might hinder your sleep

What and when we eat or drink can also make it harder to get a good night's sleep. Simple changes might make our sleep better.

Dinner time

Eating an evening meal too close to bedtime can affect how well we sleep. Having a gap of 2-3 hours between your last meal and going to bed can be very helpful.

As we get older, our digestion slows down. This varies a lot between people and can depend on how active they are. For some people, switching their largest meal to the middle of the day or having it earlier in the evening can be helpful.

A large gap after your final meal may result in feeling a little hungry so a small snack can be helpful to avoid hunger disrupting your sleep (see the previous section).

What's on the menu?

Some meals can be less favourable for sleep. Spicy or fatty foods, we sometimes use the term 'rich' or 'heavy' food, can make it harder to sleep if eaten too late in the evening. Eating meals like these a little earlier can help. The amount of food can also interfere with sleep. Although a large meal can make us feel very sleepy, (think of that sleepy lull post-Christmas dinner), going to bed after a large meal can cause poorer sleep through indigestion and discomfort.

What we drink and when

If you are getting up in the night to empty your bladder, reducing how much you drink in the evenings may help. It's important to compensate earlier in the day by front-loading your fluid intake to avoid dehydration, as you may wake up with a dry mouth and feeling thirsty.

There are some drinks that we need to consider more specifically:

- Caffeinated drinks - Caffeine stimulates the nervous system and makes us more alert which makes it harder to fall asleep. The effects of caffeine can last several hours after consuming it. Simply switching to decaf or non-caffeinated drinks after lunchtime can make a big difference.

- Alcohol - It is easy to think that alcohol helps you sleep. It can be easier to fall asleep after a few drinks and we may feel like we slept very deeply. Alcohol actually interferes with our sleep. We don't fall into the same sleeping pattern associated with refreshing and restful sleep, leaving us more likely to feel groggy in the morning. It's best to stick to the UK's low risk drinking guidelines (see the Hot Flushes chapter).

Sleep hygiene and further information

Practicing good sleep hygiene is really important. For practical information on ways to help you sleep better, check out the factsheet from Women's Health Concern called Menopause and Insomnia on our Links and Resources page.

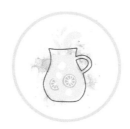

Healthy Hydration

Talking about the last great taboo – how to avoid becoming a 'leaky lady'

Why can hydration get tricky in menopause?

We all know how important hydration is for health. It can be easy not to drink enough especially when we are busy, physically active or in hotter weather. There is one thing that menopausal women find challenging which can make keeping well hydrated harder. Something that no one likes to talk about.

Many women find that their bladder becomes a little controlling – demanding to be emptied more often or to be emptied multiple times in the night. These demands can be extremely urgent and not to mention the leakiness especially when jumping around. Seen as a normal part of aging, becoming noticeable through menopause, women often manage the inconvenience and shrug it off – even when the symptoms become a source of stress or impact their sleep significantly.

These issues often cause women to subconsciously or actively manage their fluid intake in a way that results in drinking less overall. Waking up regularly through the night to empty your bladder is going to naturally cause you to drink less before you go to bed. Although this has been shown to help, the downside is that the reduction in fluid intake is often not compensated for.

In the day time, the need to empty your bladder more frequently can become inconvenient for commuting, working or other daily tasks. Women can then try to manage this by avoiding drinking at certain times. The aim is to reduce the inconvenient toilet trips, especially when there might not be access to one. Once again, this reduction in fluid intake may not be compensated for, especially for women who are out and about a lot or in jobs that make toilet trips difficult.

The importance of hydration in menopause

Drinking less may in the short-term seem to help manage the inconvenience but the effect on hydration is not good for health and well-being. This is true for anyone. Water makes up a large proportion of our body weight (about 60% on average), (Benelam & Wyness, 2010) and it is fundamental to the chemical processes that make our body work. Even mild dehydration can impact how well we think and how we feel – often before we feel any signs of thirst.

Many of the feelings and effects of poor hydration affect us in ways often associated with menopausal symptoms. Here are some examples:

- Dehydration affects clarity of thought and judgement – exacerbating brain fog.
- It can leave us feeling low in energy or tired which can affect our mood, all of which may already be impacted by menopause.
- Poor hydration can result in drier skin which is often a problem for menopausal women.
- It can cause headaches which are often more common for menopausal women.
- Being well hydrated helps us to manage changes in body temperature therefore dehydration may exacerbate hot flushes or night sweats.
- It can increase the risk of urinary tract infections and bladder dysfunction.

Staying well hydrated helps your muscles work more efficiently. Activity is harder if you are dehydrated and you can feel that you have less energy. Don't forget that your heart is also a muscle so hydration is important to help the heart do its job. Hydration is important for heart health.

It is really important to note that poor hydration makes us more at risk of urinary tract infections and bladder dysfunction. Women are becoming dehydrated trying to manage bladder symptoms but in doing so are aggravating the symptoms they are trying to manage.

Dehydration results in strong concentrated urine which irritates the bladder. This increases urgency and frequency, and may also cause discomfort.

If you are suffering from urgency or discomfort when emptying your bladder it is important to see your doctor. These symptoms can be a sign of infection or other bladder issues, especially if there is any trace of blood in the urine.

Urgency and discomfort can be aggravated by certain foods and drinks. Alcohol (some drinks are more irritating than others), coffee (both caffeinated and decaf), some soft drinks (the more acidic the more irritating), some fruits, spicy foods, some strong cheeses (including blue cheese) are all examples of foods that can be problematic. The degree to which foods irritate a sensitive bladder is very personal and is more intense if you are dehydrated. A bladder diary that records foods and drinks, and the degree of the symptoms can give some insight.

The effect of menopause on bladder control

Bladder issues increase with age however this is more marked in women and there seems to be an increase that coincides with menopause. Oestrogen directly affects our pelvic area and the loss of its impact as we go through menopause has an effect on the bladder and continence issues.

The vagina becomes drier and changes in a way that reduces the protection it offers the urethra from irritation and infection. The pelvic floor, including in women who have not had children, slackens which impacts the bladder. We know that nocturia improves with topical, vaginal oestrogen and may also improve other bladder issues.

Stress and anxiety can stimulate the bladder nerves. There does seem to be an effect of serotonin on bladder function and some women respond well to Selective Serotonin Reuptake Inhibitors – medication used for depression. If we consider the chapters that discuss the effect of hormones on serotonin then it may be that any lifestyle factors that improve these symptoms may also be positive too for bladder function, but this is yet to be explored.

There is a false sense that a weakening bladder is a part of ageing as a woman, and even more so for women who have had children – something for which there is little that can be done – when in most cases there are treatment options that can cure or significantly reduce the problem.

When these problems start to appear they can be managed and worked around. Slowly, they can become more than an inconvenience. These symptoms can eventually be a severe limitation on quality of life, impact your health in ways you may not expect and even be the reason, in later years, that result in your loss of independence.

Incontinence is not just inconvenient

We have already seen that bladder issues can impair sleep and make it harder to stay hydrated. Going to the toilet more frequently can get in the way of life and be annoying and inconvenient. It may be a bit stressful if you start to worry about a little accident, but it doesn't kill you. Does it?

Bladder issues often stop women from exercising. The fear of a little accident can stop women going for a run or joining an exercise class. It also reduces the length of walks or time spent active, out and about, for fear of being caught short. This has an impact on both heart and bone health.

For similar reasons, women often stop doing some things they enjoy, or meeting friends, if it means they might cause inconvenience to others or potential embarrassment – not sharing a car journey or sitting in a cinema. It can cause stress at work when doing presentations or important events or meetings. It may impact the choice of clothes, holidays or days out based on the chances of being caught without a toilet when it is needed. This can result in isolation and feeling low.

Depression and significant bladder problems often go hand in hand with stress aggravating symptoms. As it is something that is often uncomfortable to be candid and open about, women often suffer in silence.

Worse still, as women get older, rushing to the toilet can get harder. Looking into the future, as this is also about health well beyond menopause, falls that result in fracture are often the result of rushing to the toilet. This could lead to a loss of independence.

Ignoring bladder issues can lead to more than just the occasional need for an incontinence pad and poorer sleep (although we know that poor sleep is detrimental to health). It can really become far more impactful on life.

This doesn't have to happen. If you have bladder issues, speak to a doctor. Take a bladder diary with you. So often the right referral or the right medication, which may include HRT, can reduce or solve the problem, helping you to live a healthier and safer post-menopausal life. We need to be comfortable talking about it and asking for support sooner rather than later.

Hydration advice for menopause

General advice is the same for everyone – most of us should aim to drink 1.5 - 2 litres of fluid a day. If active, or if the weather is particularly hot, then it is important to drink more.

If you are tapering how much you drink to help reduce night time toilet trips or to manage other bladder symptoms be sure to compensate for the times of day you are drinking less.

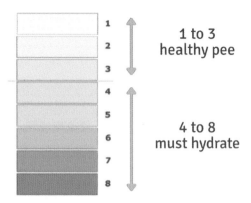

The colour of our urine can give an indication of how hydrated we are. Urine should be a light straw colour - colours 1-3. Darker urine indicates a need to hydrate.

It can be surprisingly easy to inadvertently become dehydrated. This can have an impact on menopausal symptoms in addition to the effects of dehydration on well-being and health experienced by everyone.

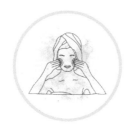

Healthy Hair, Skin and Eyes

Can diet stop menopausal hair loss and my skin and eyes becoming dry?

Hair, skin and eyes

Many women report significant hair loss post-menopause and that their skin and eyes become drier and more sensitive. These things can be hard to manage. There are many supplements, dietary changes and products available to older women claiming to stop these changes and improve hair, skin and eyes at this time in their lives. What's the evidence?

Hair loss

The reason behind hair loss is hormonal. Oestrogen and progesterone help hair grow faster, and the drop in these hormones during menopause is thought to lead to hair that grows slower and thinner.

The change in balance between female and male hormones at menopause means that androgen (male) hormones have a stronger effect in our bodies. Androgen hormones shrink hair follicles, contributing to hair loss on the head and cause more soft facial hairs like 'peach fuzz' or a few small sprouts of hair on the chin.

Our genes play a role in hair loss, both menopausal and due to natural ageing. If a female relative's hair has thinned after menopause you may be more likely to experience it yourself. Hair loss can be upsetting and cause anxiety, but be assured that most menopause related hair loss slows down over time.

Extreme stress, illness, or a deficiency in certain nutrients, such as iron or zinc, may also contribute to hair loss. If hair loss is accompanied by other symptoms, hair is being lost in an unusual pattern or if you have any pain or itching related to hair loss, speak to your doctor for advice.

Dry skin

The ageing of our skin is affected by our genes, the environment we are exposed to and our hormone levels. Oestrogen, in particular, has a role in growth and maintenance of tiny blood vessels within the skin. As oestrogen levels fall, blood flow in the skin is reduced. This results in thinner skin and increased water loss, which leads to dryness.

The fat in our body is redistributed during menopause, moving towards the abdomen. As a result, we lose some of the supportive fatty deposits beneath the skin of our face, neck, hands and arms. This also contributes to the thinning and drying of skin.

The thinning of the skin and the reduced fatty layer under the skin makes our skin more sensitive to the effects of the sun's rays.

As there are oestrogen receptors in the lining of the mouth, variations in hormone levels can result in a dry mouth, as well as changes to taste, an increase in dental caries and a burning sensation in the mouth among peri- and post-menopausal women. (Suri & Suri, 2014)

Skin changes can also affect the vagina, contributing to discomfort, bladder issues and the increased risk of urinary tract infections. This is covered within the Healthy Hydration chapter.

Dry eyes

The decrease in hormones during menopause can result in dry eyes. Dry eyes occur more with age and among women. Post-menopausal women are particularly prone to dry eyes. One study found almost two thirds (64%) of menopausal women, aged 45-79 years, had eye issues with the surface of their eyes such as dryness or inflammation. (Garcia-Alfaro et al., 2020)

How can diet and lifestyle help?

Healthy eating

There are a number of nutrients that have a role in skin, hair and eye health. A healthy and varied diet should provide all of them. Below are some useful foods, which provide nutrients linked to hair, skin and eye health.

Oily fish

Omega-3 fatty acids help moisturise and protect skin from sun damage and may help reduce dry eyes. (Liu & Ji, 2014) Oily fish are the best source of these beneficial omega-3 fats. These include salmon, mackerel, trout, anchovies, sardines and herring. If you don't eat fish, you can get some plant sources of omega-3 fatty acids from flaxseed, linseeds, walnuts and rapeseed oil or consider taking an omega-3 supplement.

Protein foods

Proteins act as the building blocks to all cells in the body, including skin and hair. Eating some protein foods at each meal will help the body utilise it more effectively. Protein foods include: meat, fish, eggs, dairy products, beans, lentils, tofu and soya products.

Fruit and vegetables

Including a variety of yellow, red and green leafy vegetables and yellow fruits in your diet will provide beta-carotene and carotenoids that play an important role in maintaining eye health. Vitamin C is important in the production of collagen that is important for our skin.

Iron-containing foods

Low iron levels have been linked to hair loss. Including red meat in your diet a few times a week will provide easily absorbable iron. If you don't eat meat, make sure you include plant sources of iron such as beans, peas, lentils, tofu, nuts, seeds and green leafy vegetables like spinach, kale, broccoli and fruits such as dried apricots and raisins. Some breakfast cereals are fortified with iron.

The polyphenols (tannins) in tea and coffee can hinder iron absorption from plant foods, so avoid these drinks with meals. Wait about an hour after your meal before having a brew.

Hydration

Keeping well hydrated is important for your body to function properly. Aim to drink 6-8 glasses of water a day. To check if you're hydrated enough, your urine should be a light straw colour. If you are waking up in the night to use the toilet then it may be wise to drink more in the morning and early afternoon, so that you can drink a little less in the evening to help you sleep longer. It is important not to be dehydrated, as strong urine can increase the number of trips to the toilet and the risk of urinary tract infections (see the Healthy Hydration chapter).

Collagen

Collagen gets spoken about a lot in relation to menopause and in particular in relation to skin. As we age, our collagen production falls and this may contribute to the reduction in the elasticity of our skin and the appearance of wrinkles. Skin collagen levels decrease quite rapidly in peri-menopause, by around 30% in the first 5 years, followed by a further decline of 2% per year for the next 15 years. (Zouboulis et al., 2022)

As described in the Bone Health chapter, our diet is important for collagen production. Including foods that support the production of collagen is likely to contribute to the health and appearance of our skin just as it may support bone health. A Mediterranean style diet will provide the nutrients necessary for collagen production.

Collagen production requires protein so including a range of protein foods across the day such as fish, eggs, dairy foods, soya foods, legumes, meat and nuts and seeds is important. Alongside protein, the body needs a range of micronutrients found in plant foods to turn protein into collagen, the most well-known being vitamin C.

 Severe vitamin C deficiency is the cause of scurvy which is visible by the body's connective tissue essentially falling apart.

Reducing the amount of processed foods may also support the skin. Compounds found in foods such as processed meat like hot dogs and bacon, fried foods like French fries and roasted or grilled meats can accumulate in the skin. To give them their scientific name, advanced glycation end products (AGEs) are harmful compounds that can cause collagen to stiffen and inactivate proteins responsible for collagen repair.

Smoking and too much alcohol are both associated with poorer skin condition. This may be because they both interfere with collagen production.

Collagen supplements are often marketed for reduction in wrinkles and better skin. We discuss these in the Myths and Marketing chapter.

Other factors

Exercise

Regular exercise has numerous benefits for health and well-being during menopause. For our skin, keeping active helps improve circulation, which is likely to benefit skin health.

Sun protection

Post-menopausal skin is more sensitive to the sun's ultraviolet light, which can damage the collagen and elastin, which keep your skin smooth and supple. Too much sun exposure can increase wrinkles and dry our skin. Wearing sunscreen can help lessen the damage. Sunscreen blocks the rays that stimulate the skin's production of vitamin D. If you always wear sunscreen or always wear clothes that cover your skin, it is even more important to remember to take a vitamin D supplement.

Eye protection

Limiting screen time and protecting your eyes from the strong sunlight can help protect your eyes. Avoiding potential irritants to eyes such as smoke, pollen and some contact lenses is likely to benefit your eyes. Some eye drops may also be useful to help relieve dry eyes, so ask your doctor or pharmacist for advice.

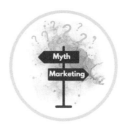

Myths and Marketing

Supplements and diets for menopause - do they deliver what they promise?

Information overload

Menopause is finally becoming more spoken about and is less taboo. With the increase in political and media attention, menopausal women have become an even bigger target group for marketing and unsubstantiated information.

Motivated by a set of issues affecting their quality of life and future long-term health, this group are researching solutions and are open to trying them. As many women approaching and post menopause have more disposable income, they are willing to invest in better health and well-being. There is a mountain of information, tips and products vying for their attention and hard-earned cash. How can we possibly sort the useful from the marketing and myths?

Supplements

Supplements for menopausal symptoms abound and can be either nutritional supplements or herbal remedies. Here we consider the difference between these two groups of supplements and a few of the most commonly advocated.

Food and nutritional supplements

There are a multitude of nutritional supplements targeted at older and menopausal women. In legal terms, they are considered foods even though they are often sold in pharmacies. They have to adhere to food safety and health claims legislation.

While a nutrient may have a beneficial effect taken as a supplement, most nutrients can have adverse effects at higher doses. With the variety of supplements available, often highlighting different potential benefits, it may be tempting for women to take more than one supplement. It can be easy to double-up on nutrients. A multivitamin, marketed for menopause, may contain nutrients contained in another supplement.

In general, eating a wide variety of foods with the aim of obtaining nutrients from your diet should be the focus. There are many components in our food that we do not fully understand. It is clear that there are interactions between components which increase the benefit of the nutrients in our food. These benefits are lost when taking nutrients in supplemental form.

Some common food and nutritional supplements marketed to menopausal women are summarised here:

Magnesium supplements

Magnesium plays many important roles throughout the body. It is an essential nutrient in all human tissues, particularly your bones. Magnesium is involved in obtaining energy from food and also plays a role in muscle and nerve function and blood clotting. It is important in making serotonin and therefore is often connected with sleep and mood. Your body uses more magnesium when stressed, as it helps soothe the nervous system, which is why it is often taken for managing anxiety.

The amount of magnesium an adult woman needs is 270mg a day. Although deficiency of magnesium is rare, it is quite common for adults to have low levels. You should be able to get all the magnesium you need from your diet by including a variety of foods including green leafy vegetables, nuts, legumes, wholegrain cereals, dairy foods, meat and fish.

Although evidence is not conclusive, you may want to try a supplement containing magnesium to see if you feel any benefit in relation to improved mood, reduced anxiety or better sleep. Too much magnesium (supplements of more than 400mg) can cause diarrhea.

Omega-3 supplements

Omega-3 polyunsaturated fatty acids are essential for health. They include alpha-linolenic acid (ALA), a short-chain omega-3, found in plant foods such as hemp, chia seeds, pumpkin seeds, walnuts and rapeseed oil. The longer-chain omega-3s, known as eicosapentaenoic acid (EPA) and docosahexaenoic acid (DHA), are found in oily fish and egg yolk.

EPA and DHA are particularly beneficial for heart health, brain function and eye health. The body can convert short-chain omega-3 into longer-chain omega-3s but it's not very efficient at doing so. Dietary recommendations for EPA and DHA range from 250mg to 500mg daily. This amount can be obtained by eating two portions of fish a week, including one portion of an oily-fish.

An omega-3 supplement containing EPA and DHA can be beneficial, especially if you don't eat oily fish.

Omega-3 may help alleviate night sweats, although there appears to be no benefit in reducing hot flushes or improving sleep quality. (Mohammady et al., 2018) There is a need for more research in this area, as only a few studies have been carried out.

A fish oil supplement will also contain vitamins A and D. Both these vitamins are found in multivitamin supplements so it is important to be sure that you are not taking too much. High levels of vitamin A are not advised in post-menopausal women as it may have a negative effect on bone health.

Phytoestrogens (isoflavones and lignans) supplements

Plant-based oestrogens, or phytoestrogens, are found in plants. The two main types are isoflavones (found mainly in soybeans and soya products such as tofu, although very small amounts are also found in lentils and chickpeas) and lignans (found in linseed or flaxseed, sesame seeds, wholegrains, fruits and vegetables).

Phytoestrogens have a mild oestrogen-like effect in humans, when consumed in the diet regularly in sufficient amounts. Some studies have shown that phytoestrogens may be useful in relieving menopausal symptoms, particularly hot flushes. (Messina et al., 2022) It can take a few months for the benefits of phytoestrogens to be felt. It may be more effective to consume foods with plant oestrogens several times a day, rather than one larger dose.

Whilst including foods with phytoestrogens in your diet may be useful for managing menopausal symptoms, more studies are needed to confirm whether isoflavone supplements are safe and effective in reducing menopausal symptoms. More research is needed to understand the role that phytoestrogens may have in breast and ovarian cancer risk, particularly if consumed in high doses or in combination with HRT. It is best to seek medical advice before consuming high-dose phytoestrogen supplements.

A diet rich in plant-based foods makes a good contribution to a range of phytoestrogens and it's thought that the levels consumed from foods are unlikely to pose a risk. Getting phytoestrogens from foods will also provide a healthy range of other nutrients as these foods tend provide fibre, vitamins and minerals as well as being naturally rich in protein and low in saturated fat.

Collagen supplements

There are a lot of collagen supplements on the market and some of these are marketed to menopausal women. Collagen is a protein naturally produced in our body. As we get older our body produces less of it. Since collagen is the main protein in connective tissue, it is touted as the supplement of choice to maintain healthy skin, joints and bones for menopausal women. What does the evidence say?

Joint health

Collagen is the main protein in tendons, bones, ligaments and cartilage and its thought that collagen supplementation may support joint health and reduce joint pain. There is some evidence that collagen supplements may improve joint stiffness in osteoarthritis. (Garcia-Coronado et al., 2019) Other evidence that supports this shows that supplementing collagen along with vitamin C may be beneficial in those who have a low intake of this vitamin. (Shaw et al., 2017) Vitamin C is needed for collagen production. More good quality studies are still needed in this area.

Bone health

Evidence shows that supplementing women who are at risk of osteoporosis with the specific peptides present in collagen (5g of collagen specific peptides), increases bone mineral density. (Konig et al. , 2018) A follow-up study in a small number of those women confirmed these findings. (Zdzieblik et al., 2021)

Skin health

The use of collagen supplements to support skin health has recently been gaining popularity. Collagen helps keep skin strong and elastic.

Some studies have shown that taking collagen supplements may improve skin hydration and elasticity and help reduce wrinkles. (de Miranda et al., 2021) However, these studies tend to be funded by companies producing collagen products. It's also difficult to determine whether the study results were due to collagen or some of the other ingredients contained within the supplements, or any lifestyle habits of the participants.

The evidence that collagen supplements provide skin benefits are not as strong as for other factors. There is stronger evidence that using sunscreen, not smoking and eating a healthy, balanced diet is beneficial for supporting skin health. (Krutmann et al., 2017)

Safe and effective?

Collagen supplements are generally considered to be safe. There is very little evidence of harm in taking collagen as a supplement, however collagen supplements, especially when marketed for specific purposes, often contain other nutrients or ingredients. Be aware that they may be present in other supplements you take resulting in higher doses than are safe. Additional ingredients may not be suitable for you.

Collagen that you consume either from dietary sources such as meat, fish and bone broth or from collagen supplements isn't absorbed as collagen to be used directly as collagen in our bodies. Like any other protein we consume, it is broken down and absorbed as amino acids (the building blocks of protein). The body then uses the amino acids to create whichever protein it needs most. It has been argued that collagen is no more effective in benefitting skin than adequate dietary protein intake. (Spiro & Locker, 2018)

Although there may be some benefits of collagen supplements, focusing on eating a wide variety of good quality protein foods across the day as part of a healthy balanced diet is likely to be more beneficial for your skin, health and finances.

With all supplements, we should always consider potential downsides. If you wish to try supplements do talk with your doctor or a pharmacist before making your choice.

Herbal remedies

Herbal medicines are regulated differently from pharmaceuticals, vitamin and mineral supplements. They are not subject to the same safety or efficacy testing as pharmaceutical drugs, so you really don't know what you're getting. If something is natural it is not always safe.

It should be noted that there is limited evidence showing measurable and repeatable benefit for most people with regards to herbal products. Additionally, there are limited studies into the safety of their long-term use and of high doses.

Common herbal remedies claiming to improve menopausal symptoms

Herbal Medicine	Claimed benefits and notes
Black Cohosh rhizome and root (*Cimicifuga racemosa or Actaea racemosa*)	Research suggests Black Cohosh extracts and some combination products containing Black Cohosh may reduce hot flushes and other menopause symptoms. It's not clear if Black Cohosh is safe for women who have had hormone-sensitive conditions such as breast cancer. (NIH, 2020)
Sage (*Salvia officinalis or Salvia lavandulaefolia*)	For relief from excessive sweating associated with the menopause (MHRA, 2022) although very little research has been done on it. Some species of Sage contain a compound called thujone which may negatively impact the nervous system when taken in too-large amounts or for too long. (NIH, 2020)
St. John's Wort (*Hypericum perforatum*)	For relief of symptoms of the menopause including hot flushes, night sweats, slightly low mood and mild anxiety, based on traditional use only. St John's Wort can weaken the effects of many medicines, including antidepressants and birth control pills. (NIH, 2020)
Peony Root (*Paeonia lactiflora L.*)	For the symptomatic relief of menopausal hot flushes, based on traditional use only.
Red clover (*Trifolium pratense*)	Red Clover contains isoflavones, compounds that are structurally similar to oestrogen. It has been promoted for reducing hot flushes and osteoporosis, but the evidence is inconsistent. (NIH, 2020) It has also been suggested to have a beneficial effect on cholesterol levels, although further studies are needed as evidence is very limited. (Kanadys et al, 2020)
Ginseng (*Ginseng Panax*)	For alleviating menopausal hot flushes and improving quality of life, however, good quality studies are limited. (Lee et al., 2022) Insomnia is the herb's most common side effect. Ginseng may interact with certain medications. (NIH, 2020)
Evening Primrose Oil (*Oenothera biennis*)	Although it's widely used and well-tolerated by most people, there's insufficient scientific evidence to show whether evening primrose oil is helpful for the relief of menopause symptoms. (NIH, 2020)
Flaxseed and Flaxseed oil (*Linum usitatissimum*)	Studies have had mixed results on whether flaxseed helps with symptoms of menopause. (NIH, 2020) Flaxseed and Flaxseed oil supplements seem to be well tolerated in limited amounts and few side effects have been reported. Like any fibre supplement, it should be taken with plenty of water. (NIH, 2020)

Looking for products with Traditional Herbal Registration Certification or the THR mark gives some assurance that the product has been produced safely. To use the THR mark on a herbal product, and make claims relating to its traditional or historical use, the Medicines and Healthcare products Regulatory Agency (MHRA) must be happy with scientific data on the sourcing and quality of the product as well as safety data and evidence on the traditional use of the product supplied by the brand. A THR mark however, doesn't mean the product is completely safe for everyone to take.

Many herbals recommended for menopausal women relate to the effect of the herbal on sleep, anxiety and mood with the assumption that the findings seen in non-menopausal groups can be carried over to those symptoms as they appear as a product of menopause – this assumption may not be valid. Many herbals are used in combination in the form of a 'multi-botanical', of which there is even less science to support efficacy and safety. (Stacie and Studee, 2005)

Herbal remedies may interact with prescription medicines. For example, St John's Wort can interact with antidepressants and a range of other medications and decrease the effectiveness of HRT or oral contraceptives. If you are going to try traditional herbal remedies, have a chat with your doctor first, particularly if you take other medication.

Special diets and claims about foods

In the pages of many women's magazines and on social media there are diets and tips on what you should and shouldn't eat if you are going through the menopause. Any diet that advocates extremes or cuts out whole food groups is likely to have a downside.

Completely plant-based diets

Some articles claim a completely plant-based diet is best, yet we know a vegan diet may put women at greater risk of osteoporosis. (Tong et al. , 2020) If you choose to follow a vegan diet it's important to plan your food carefully and consider taking supplements, not just for bone health, to ensure you are not missing out on important nutrients. Nutrients important for brain, mood and heart health can also be reduced when consuming a diet completely free from animal products.

Keto diets

The keto diet is widely touted as beneficial for weight management and to support menopause, despite being regularly highlighted by nutrition professionals as a diet with many downsides. The keto diet was developed for children with epilepsy who do not respond to medication.

Keto is an extreme diet, which requires eliminating most carbohydrates from the diet. The fibre compounds that keep our gut microbiome healthy are also eliminated. As outlined previously in this book, gut health plays an important part in managing menopause symptoms and related health issues.

Tryptophan, that is so important for mood, sleep and other aspects of brain function, is better absorbed and utilised in the presence of carbohydrates. The brain can only use glucose, a carbohydrate, for energy. The limiting of carbohydrates can induce 'brain fog' or feeling fuzzy headed. A Keto diet can result in feeling tired and fatigued. All of these side effects could amplify menopausal symptoms rather than help.

The no-sugar diet

Whilst it is healthy to reduce the amount of sugary foods and sugar-sweetened drinks we consume, there is no evidence that completely cutting out sugar altogether is helpful for menopausal symptoms.

Many 'sugar-free' recipes or 'natural sugar replacements' are sugars in another form. Artificial sweeteners can be intensely sweet so do not help us to move away from sweet flavours and emerging evidence suggests that some may have a negative effect on our microbiome. (Suez et al., 2022)

Healthier 'guilt-free' bakes are often just as high in calories, fats and sugars as their equivalents, sometimes even higher. They are often far more expensive and may not taste as good.

Intermittent fasting

Intermittent fasting, such as alternate-day fasting, the 5:2 diet, and time-restricted eating, is certainly a big topic. There is no doubt that for some people a shift in eating pattern to eat only between certain hours or moving a main meal to earlier in the day brings positive outcomes, however the evidence does not support this as a recommendation for all.

There are some potential downsides for some people. During periods of fasting people can feel unwell or get headaches. Fasting can lead to an overall reduction in nutrients in a negative way or eating poorly during the hours that eating is permitted so there is no overall improvement in nutrition.

Very few studies have looked at the impact of intermittent fasting on reproductive hormones and no studies have been carried out so far on the impact of intermittent fasting in peri- or post-menopausal women. (Cienfuegos et al., 2022)

Hormone balancing diet

There are diets that imply that they can modify your hormones and manage menopause alone. Whilst eating well provides the components your body needs to produce your hormones effectively, diet cannot replace or alter your hormone levels. It can only optimise what your body is doing. Menopause and the dropping of oestrogen is a natural process – eating well may ease the process but it cannot replace human oestrogen.

Diets that describe different types of bodies or hormone types are describing the different ways that our bodies respond to the change in hormone balance. There is no evidence that a particular diet is best for different hormone types. The advice is the same for all women. Follow the principles of a Mediterranean diet, look after your gut health and include some phytoestrogen containing foods.

 Exercise, yoga and mindfulness meditation are all complementary or alternative therapies that are generally low risk, low cost and are accessible options worth trying. In addition to supporting healthy menopause, they can also support overall health and well-being. Some of these can be done with friends and this can add further benefits.

Making the right choice for you

Ultimately, the choice is yours alone. We are all different and we have to come to the best decision for our own bodies. Science may not have all the answers and if something gives you relief whilst doing you no harm or breaking the bank then test it out. But before trying something new, ask yourself some questions:

What is your inner sceptic saying?

If something sounds too good to be true it often is. Who is telling you and how might they benefit? Are they qualified and, if so, what does that qualification mean? Find an independent opinion and seek out balanced discussions with the pros and cons.

What is the evidence?

Some of the claims made for supplements, herbal products and specific diets on menopause and its symptoms are lacking evidence. Appreciate that anecdotal evidence is often solely opinion, not fact. Something may appear to benefit someone else, they may feel very strongly about the effect of a diet or supplement – it does not automatically follow that it will work for you too. Their story may feel very true, and may indeed be true, but there is no control group and those who found no effect do not tend to speak up so loudly.

This doesn't mean that you shouldn't try something where the evidence is weak. As said above, science does not yet have all the answers. But do be sure that you are not doing yourself any harm. Anything you try must, as a minimum, do no harm. That includes putting a large dent in your wallet for no proven gain if this means you then cannot afford to do things that are known to give you health benefits.

What are the risks to me?

Everyone is different in terms of health conditions, allergies, medications and genetics. Before you try anything new it is worth talking to your doctor. Pharmacists are also knowledgeable about interactions between drugs, herbal remedies and supplements. Ask questions.

If a supplement, diet or herbal remedy doesn't work then stop. If they make you feel unwell or strange then stop. Whatever you might read or hear about other people's stories, one person's medicine can be another's poison.

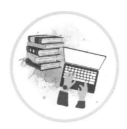

Links and Resources

Where can I find evidence based information on managing menopause?

Want to find out more?

There is so much more information on all aspects of menopause beyond food and diet that we haven't included in this book. Below is a list of resources and links that come from trusted sources.

General menopause and health information	
The Menopause Charity	www.themenopausecharity.org
Womens Health Concern	www.womens-health-concern.org
Menopause Matters	www.menopausematters.co.uk
Manage My Menopause	www.managemymenopause.co.uk
Rock My Menopause	www.rockmymenopause.com
Daisy Network	www.daisynetwork.org
British Dietetic Association	www.bda.uk.com/resource/menopause-diet.html
British Nutrition Foundation	www.nutrition.org.uk/life-stages/women/menopause
Better Health: Drink Less	www.nhs.uk/better-health/drink-less
Women Positively Aging (podcast)	www.alo-solutions.com/podcasts/women-positively-ageing
Dr Louise Newson (podcast)	https://thedrlouisenewsonpodcast.podbean.com

Links on specific topics

Bone health

British Dietetic Association. Osteoporosis and diet: Food Fact Sheet	www.bda.uk.com/resource/osteoporosis-diet.html
Royal Osteoporosis Society	www.theros.org.uk

Heart health

British Nutrition Foundation	www.nutrition.org.uk/health-conditions/heart-disease-and-stroke/
Heart UK UCLP© and the Menopause	www.heartuk.org.uk/ultimate-cholesterol-lowering-plan/uclp-menopause
NHS Heart Age Calculator	www.nhs.uk/conditions/nhs-health-check/check-your-heart-age-tool/

Sleep

Women's Health Concern Fact Sheet on Menopause and insomnia	www.womens-health-concern.org/help-and-advice/factsheets/menopause-and-insomnia
NHS: Insomnia Information	www.nhs.uk/conditions/insomnia

Mood

American Gut Project (2018)	The American Gut Health Project - Big Data from World's Largest Citizen Science Microbiome Project Serves Food for Thought.
British Dietetic Association. Food and mood: Food Fact Sheet	www.bda.uk.com/resource/food-facts-food-and-mood.html
Mind website	www.mind.org.uk

Bladder issues

Elaine Miller, Pelvic Physiotherapist	www.gussetgrippers.co.uk
NHS: What are pelvic floor exercises?	www.nhs.uk/common-health-questions/womens-health/what-are-pelvic-floor-exercises/

Hair loss

Women's Health Concern Fact Sheet on Menopausal hair loss	www.womens-health-concern.org/help-and-advice/factsheets/menopausal-hair-loss

Hormone Replacement Therapy

NHS: Overview of HRT	www.nhs.uk/conditions/hormone-replacement-therapy-hrt

Recipes

Ideas to put some of the advice into practice

A range of recipes for all times of the day

I n this book there is lots of talk of nutrients and foods that contribute to a balanced diet to support good health throughout menopause and beyond. Incorporating the advice into menus can sometimes be hard. We have pulled together a range of recipes including breakfast ideas, light meals, snacks and dinner options that embrace the advice in the book.

What kind of recipes are included?

You will see that the recipes include lots of plant-based ingredients and aim to be rich in fibre to support a healthy gut. If you currently don't eat lots of plants and fibre-rich foods, eating lots of these recipes close together might make you feel a little bloated or uncomfortable, particularly if you are not hydrated. Introducing lots of fibre and new plant foods too quickly doesn't allow your gut microbes to adjust.

There are protein-rich breakfasts and snacks to help to spread protein intake throughout the day using a range of protein-rich foods. With bone health in mind, we have recipes with calcium-rich foods and foods containing vitamin D.

The recipes also include foods with a range of healthy fats that support heart and brain health. We have chosen recipes that are lower in saturated fat or help to support good cholesterol management.

We have also chosen simple recipes, some very quick and some that could be batch-cooked to provide a meal another day. Also, we haven't forgotten a few sweet things because sometimes that is just the thing we need.

ENJOY!

Mini Salmon Frittatas

Ready in **30 minutes** • Serves **12 mini frittatas**

Breakfast is often the meal we eat that is lowest in protein. The science says that spreading protein across the day has lots of benefits for maintaining muscle. Eggs for breakfast is a great option but often we don't have time to whip up something cooked before heading out for the day. These frittatas provide a great start to the day as they have a range of B-vitamins which help reduce tiredness and fatigue.

These mini frittatas can be waiting in the fridge or freezer for you. They can be quickly reheated whilst making some wholemeal, seeded or sourdough toast adding fibre to support good gut health.

These frittatas include some oily fish and vegetables but don't be confined to salmon and spinach. You could add a range of different tasty ingredients.

Frittatas are also a great option for a packed lunch as they can be eaten cold. Have them as a light meal with salad or steamed veggies and potatoes.

Nutrition per serving (2 mini frittatas):

240 cals • 14 g fat (3.9 g saturates) • 2.6 g carbs (1.1 g total sugars)
0.5 g fibre • 25 g protein • 1.2 g salt

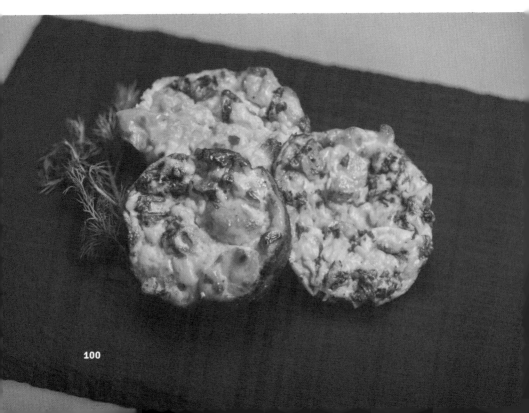

Ingredients

12 medium eggs

Black pepper (to your taste)

2 handfuls of chopped spinach

2 spring onions finely sliced

200 g hot smoked salmon or tinned salmon or precooked filet of salmon flaked

1-2 tbsp low-fat cream cheese or ricotta – you could choose one with herbs or garlic added

Fresh or frozen chives or dill

* Oil spray, for greasing muffin tin

Preparation

1. Preheat the oven to 180 °C/fan 160 °C/gas mark 4.

2. Spray a 12-hole muffin tray with oil.

3. Whisk the eggs. Add black pepper if you wish.

4. Stir through the vegetables, salmon and cheese.

5. Pour into the muffin tray, dividing equally.

6. Bake 18-20 minutes.

You can pour the mix into a greased cake tin or quiche dish. Cook for a little longer, then cut into wedges.

If you use silicone cases or trays there's no need to grease them.

They can be reheated from frozen for an easy breakfast or can be kept in the fridge for a couple of days.

Other additions include: sweetcorn, mushrooms or frozen mixed vegetables. You could swap the cheese for a blue cheese - a small amount adds lots of flavour.

Other simple egg breakfasts

Eggs can be quickly poached in a small frying pan of water, perfect on toast with microwaved tomatoes with a little olive oil and herbs.

Liven up scrambled eggs with a sprinkle of herbs, some spinach or go more Indian-style with some turmeric and garam masala.

Chop a thin omelette into a warm wrap with toppings of your choice, for example: chopped peppers, tomatoes, grated cheese, salsa, guacamole, or lower-fat crème fraiche.

Wholesome Banana Pancakes

Ready in **20 minutes** • Makes about **6 pancakes**

Pancakes may seem like a bit of an extravagant breakfast – or more of a lazy weekend brunch. By making the mixture the night before or reheating pre-made pancakes from frozen or from the fridge these can be a quick and filling breakfast. Everyone in the house will love them!

By using wholemeal flour, ground almonds and oats they have extra fibre taking you a little closer to the daily 30 g of fibre recommended for a healthy gut. The almonds also add a little extra protein. This all makes these pancakes a little more filling compared to regular pancakes.

If you like, add some soya to your day by swapping the milk for a soya alternative. No one will notice the difference in taste - great if you are not yet converted to soya products. The sweetness comes from the banana and contributes to your 5-a-day, especially if you serve the pancakes with some extra fruit.

Nutrition per pancake:

170 cals • 7.2 g fat (1.1 g saturates) • 19 g carbs (5.8 g total sugars)

2.7 g fibre • 6 g protein • 0.08 g salt

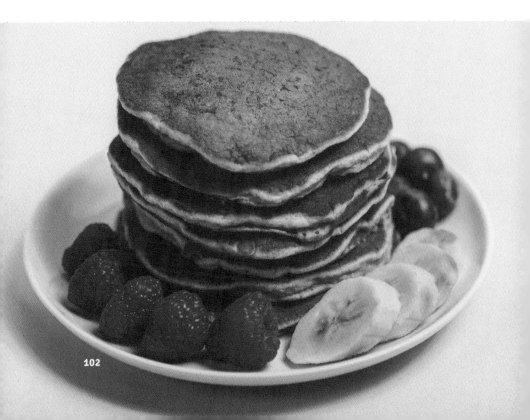

Ingredients

100 g wholemeal flour

2 tbsp almond flour

20 g oats

2 tsp baking powder

1 egg (medium), lightly beaten

240 mls milk (or soya alternative)

1 medium mashed ripe banana

1 tbsp canola/rapeseed or olive oil

Preparation

1. Mix the dry ingredients together in a bowl.

2. Add the mashed banana, egg, milk and oil and mix until just combined.

3. Heat your frying pan or griddle to a medium heat - a heavy based pan is the best - wipe it with a little oil if the pan is not non-stick.

4. When the pan is hot, pour a ladle of batter onto the pan. When bubbles start to form on the surface, flip to cook the other side. Each side should take about 3-4 minutes and should be golden.

5. Serve with fruit and yoghurt or nut butter.

Make in advance and freeze. They can be reheated from frozen in the microwave or toaster for a quick breakfast.

If you prefer lighter pancakes, use half and half plain and wholemeal flour.

To add fermented food to your breakfast, serve the pancakes with a spoonful of live yoghurt.

Stir in some frozen blueberries or raspberries to the batter.

Or, pour a spoonful of batter into the pan and drop slices of fruit into the batter, flip the pancake to brown the fruit. This works well with pineapple rings, slices of apple or banana.

Kefir Carrot Cake Overnight Oats

Ready overnight **10 minutes prep** • Serves **2**

Overnight oats have become quite a trendy breakfast. The internet is full of recipes. This recipe is inspired by carrot cake flavours. The carrot, nuts and raisins add to the fibre from the oats supporting both gut and heart health.

Prepared in advance, they can be made in a jar to be taken for a breakfast 'on-the-go' straight from the fridge. The fruit, fibre and protein should help you feel fuller for longer.

Using kefir adds a fermented food to your day which supports your gut microbes. You could also use a live yoghurt of your choice instead. Alternatively, you could use a soya alternative to yoghurt to add some phytoestrogens.

Nutrition per serving:

375 cals • 13 g fat (3.8 g saturates) • 46 g carbs (19 g total sugars)

8.8 g fibre • 15 g protein • 0.2 g salt

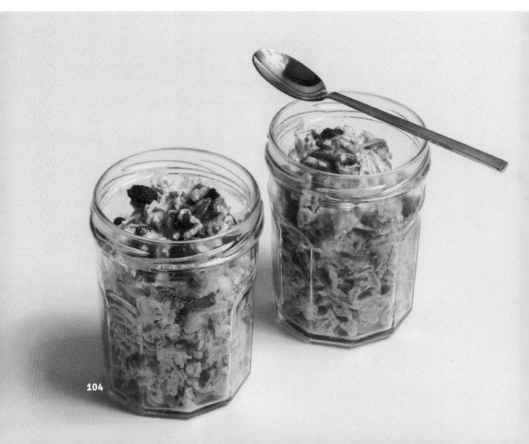

Ingredients

80 g rolled oats

1 large carrot, grated

30 g raisins

20 g chopped walnuts (or other nuts)

1 tsp ground cinnamon (to your taste)

250 mls kefir.

Preparation

1. Mix the oats, kefir, grated carrot, chopped nuts and cinnamon in a container. Leave overnight in the fridge. You could use jam jars or individual sealed pots that can be taken to work.

2. If you would like it warm then put it in the microwave for 1-2 minutes.

Prepare in individual jars to have breakfast ready-to-go.

Swap carrot for grated apple or try out other fruits - search 'overnight oats' on the internet for inspiration.

Some combinations are delicious warmed in the microwave, especially on a cold day.

Sprinkle mixed seeds to add crunch and more plant foods to feed your gut microbes.

Walnuts provide an omega-3 fatty acid called alpha-linolenic acid (ALA). Omega-3 fatty acids have an important role in heart health, brain function and reducing inflammation. Other plant foods that provide omega-3 fatty acids include flax seeds and chia seeds which also go well added to overnight oats.

Edamame Bean & Green Pea Hummus

Ready in **15 minutes** • Serves **2**

Edamame beans are young fresh soya beans so like all other soya products they are a good source of isoflavones. You can buy them frozen and ready podded making them really convenient. This beautifully green mix of edamame beans and peas makes a delicious alternative to chickpea hummus and a tasty way to add phytoestrogens to your menu.

Spread it on toast or crackers, or eat as a dip with vegetable sticks or pita bread. Not only rich in isoflavones, they are high in protein and fibre making it a filling part of a light lunch or a satisfying snack.

Nutrition per serving:

230 cals • 15 g fat (1.7 g saturates) • 8.2 g carbs (4.9 g total sugars)

7 g fibre • 12 g protein • 0.02 g salt

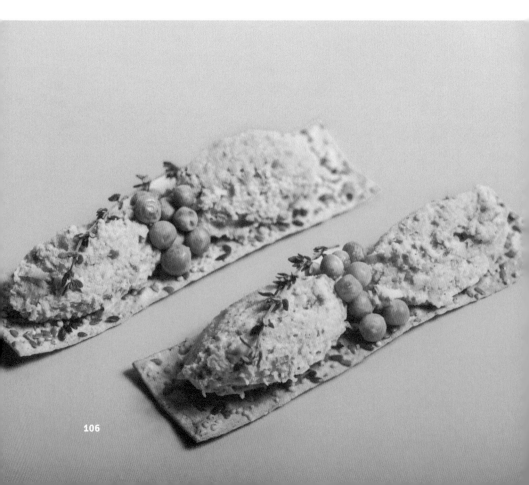

Ingredients

130 g edamame beans

100 g green peas

1 tbsp tahini

2 tbsp lemon juice (or lime juice)

Half a shallot (or a spring onion)

1 tbsp olive or rapeseed/canola oil

Freshly ground black pepper to season

Optional seasonings: chilli flakes, coriander leaves, mint leaves, garlic or parsley.

Preparation

1. Boil the edamame beans and peas for about 5 minutes until cooked. Drain and rinse under cold water to cool the beans and peas.

2. Combine the edamame beans, peas and all other ingredients except for the oil in a food processor or blender and blend until smooth.

3. Pour in oil until the mixture is a creamy texture. Add your preferred seasoning.

Try adding some cottage cheese, feta cheese or avocado.

Serve with crudités, breads or crackers - add flavour and fibre with seeded, wholegrain or rye varieties.

Turn into a sauce for pasta by stirring through some crème fraîche.

Add a sprinkle of nutritional yeast flakes - often fortified with B-vitamins and other nutrients such as zinc, iron and vitamin D, they add more than just a savoury flavour.

Roasted edamame beans can make a tasty and high-protein snack. Roast your own from fresh or frozen with seasonings that you love. If you like horseradish or mustard then try wasabi flavour.

Lentil & Tomato Salad

Ready in **10 minutes** • Serves **4**

A simple salad that is a source of fibre and high in protein that makes for a surprisingly tasty and satisfying lunch – it is perfect for a packed lunch.

You can be creative with flavours by adding herbs or a bit of chilli, a squeeze of lemon or some black pepper. Let the contents of your fridge inspire you - other crunchy salad vegetables can be added to the basics.

Nutrition per serving:

193 cals • 9.7 g fat (4.1 g saturates) • 14 g carbs (5.5 g total sugars)
3.6 g fibre • 9.5 g protein • 0.6 g salt

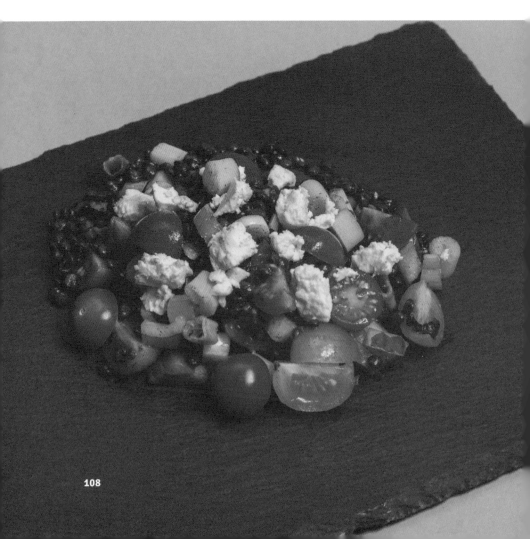

Ingredients

200 g cooked brown, green or Puy lentils – you can use a pouch or a can of pre-cooked lentils.

Half a red onion, finely diced (or you could use 1-2 spring onions).

3-4 tomatoes or a handful of cherry tomatoes.

A drizzle of olive oil – no more than 1 tbsp (or a dressing of your choice.

A little fresh or frozen herbs (parsley, chives or mint leaves work well).

100 g feta or soft fresh cheese.

A sprinkling of seeds or nuts (pumpkin seeds and pine nuts work well) (optional).

Preparation

1. Chop the tomatoes and onion.

2. Mix together in a bowl with the lentils.

3. Add oil, herbs or a dressing of your choice

4. This salad keeps well for a day or two in the fridge.

Add any crunchy vegetables to this salad - e.g. chopped peppers, celery or cucumber.

Lacking fresh vegetables? A small can of sweetcorn or vacuum-packed beetroot can add extra colour and texture.

If you're using pre-cooked lentils, choose a pack that's not too high in salt.

If you've more lentils than you need for your salad, extra can be added to other dishes like a bolognese, casserole, tagine or in our Lentil Shepherd's pie. They can also be added to gravy to serve with sausage and mash.

After the age of 40 we tend to lose muscle at a rate of around 1% each year. Lentils, and all other pulses and beans, are a great source of plant protein, which is just as effective for maintaining muscles as animal protein. Spreading protein intake across the day is important - what a good reason to try adding some pulses to a lunchtime salad.

If you have a bit of time, it's simple to prepare your own lentils. Simmer dried Puy or other dark coloured lentils in approximately three times the volume of stock. Add herbs - Herbes de Provence work well. Cook until the water has been absorbed and the lentils are soft.

Cool to use for salad, but these can also be served hot as a side dish. They compliment the Salmon with Pesto Crust very well.

Quesadillas with Refried Beans

Ready in **10 minutes** • Serves **4**

'Refried beans' is a mistranslation. The beans are not 'fried' at all. Refritos actually means recooked. A can of beans can quickly be turned into a tasty filling for quesadillas, making the traditional cheesy tortilla snack into a quick hot lunch that's high in protein, a source of fibre and includes a range of minerals that are beneficial for bone health.

The refried beans are quick to make but if you lack time to make them from scratch, you can use canned refried beans, but do beware these are higher in salt. Alternatively, simply heat some beans and mash them with a fork with a bit of seasoning for an extra quick version.

Delicious with guacamole, a little crème fraiche and salsa or a bit of salad. Wedges of quesadillas could be dunked into a bowl of hot soup on a cold day.

Nutrition per serving:

372 cals • 11 g fat (4.2 g saturates) • 46 g carbs (7.4 g total sugars)

7.5 g fibre • 19 g protein • 1.4 g salt

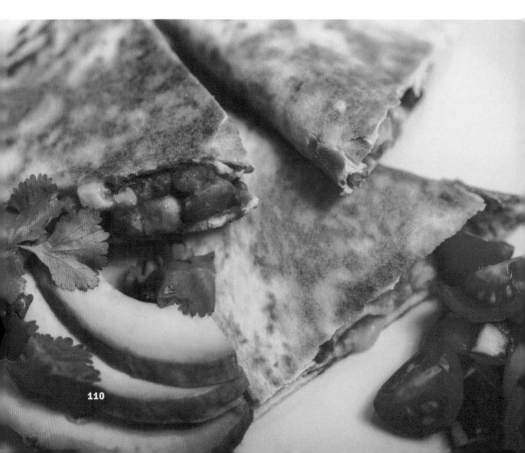

Ingredients

4 large wholemeal or multigrain or corn tortillas

100 g grated reduced-fat cheddar cheese

400 g can kidney beans

1 clove garlic, finely chopped (optional)

1 small onion, finely chopped (you could use frozen diced onions)

1 large tomato

1 tsp ground cumin

1 tsp of smoked paprika for a little spice (optional)

100 g sweetcorn

1 small red pepper, finely chopped

Spray oil

Preparation

1. Prepare your refried beans first. Heat a heavy based frying pan. Spray a little oil on the pan and soften your onion. You could also add a clove of garlic if you like.

2. Cut the tomato in half, not through the stem but around the middle, and grate the flesh into the pan. Allow to simmer for a minute. Sprinkle in your spices if you are using them

3. Add the drained beans to the pan and mash with the back of a wooden spoon or a potato masher until they are the consistency you prefer. Some like a bit of chunky texture, others prefer them smoother. When they are warmed through, put them in a bowl and keep them warm.

4. Clean the pan and put it back on the heat.

5. If it is not a non-stick pan you may need to lightly wipe it with a bit of kitchen roll soaked in a little oil or use a spray oil.

6. Place your tortilla on the hot pan.

7. Spread some refried beans on half of the tortilla and sprinkle on some finely chopped peppers and a spoonful of sweetcorn.

8. Sprinkle with some grated cheese - pick a really tasty cheddar so you won't need much and opt for a reduced-fat version. Fold the tortilla in half.

9. When the bottom of the tortilla has turned golden, flip the quesadilla.

10. When cooked on the other side, cut into wedges and serve with freshly chopped tomatoes, avocado and other salad. A little hot sauce is perfect.

Refried beans work well with any Tex Mex style meal. Serve them with fajitas, nachos and tacos. They make a delicious warm dip for potato wedges.

Use up leftover chilli in place of refried beans or buy refried beans ready made in a can.

Fridge rummage wraps - use up leftovers with the multi-fold technique.

Place a tortilla on a hot pan or prepare on a chopping board and then place in a panini or toastie maker. Cut the tortilla from the centre to the edge. In three of the quarters, place a spoonful of leftovers (e.g. chilli, refried beans, curry) in one and fill the others with suitable toppings - e.g. salsa or chutney, salad, cheese or creme fraiche. Fold on the hot pan and cook until golden and hot through. Or place in a panini or toastie maker.

Beans provide a range of vitamins and minerals and are a great combination of protein and fibre. Including a serving of 80 g of beans will count towards one of your 5-a-day and will help feed the microbes in your gut. A healthy gut microbiome has many benefits such as helping absorb nutrients from foods, maintaining a healthy weight, and possibly even improving mood.

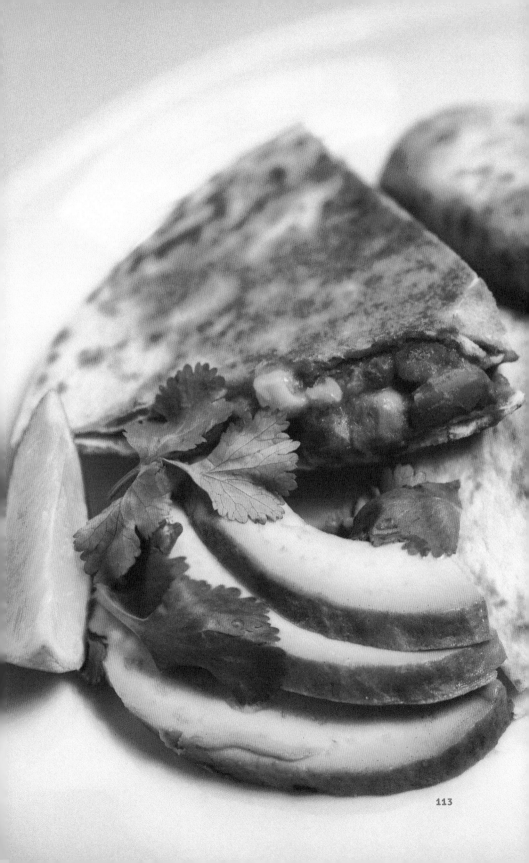

Magic Minestrone

Prepped in **10-20 minutes**, Ready in **20-30 minutes** • Serves **6**

Time can be short, life can be busy and leftovers that you thought you had can suddenly not be enough for another meal – especially if you have teenagers in the house. Tomato-based leftovers, like our Lamb Tagine recipe, can quickly be extended to a hearty soup with minimal preparation.

If you have time, you can sauté onion or leek and extra vegetables as the recipe describes but you could simply add some frozen peas, peppers, mixed vegetables or a can of sweetcorn to extend your leftovers.

As leftovers tend to taste better the next day, despite being such a quick recipe, this is always tasty. Add more herbs or spices to give it a bit extra flavour or a splash of chilli sauce.

Nutrition per serving (when made with leftover tagine):

230 cals • 5.7 g fat (1 g saturates) • 31 g carbs (9.4 g total sugars)
6.9 g fibre • 9.1 g protein • 0.3 g salt

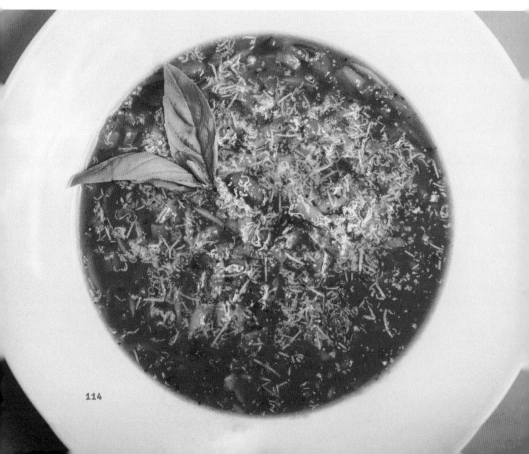

Ingredients

1 tbsp olive oil

1 onion, diced, or a leek, sliced

2 cloves garlic, sliced

1 or 2 additional vegetables (carrot, stick of celery, courgette, pepper etc)

Any tomato-based leftovers e.g. like the Lamb Tagine

400 g can of tomatoes

Freshly ground black pepper (to your taste)

400 mls stock

200 g wholemeal or high-fibre macaroni or other pasta

Preparation

1. In a soup pot, heat the olive oil. Gently fry the onion/leek and garlic.

2. Chop any extra vegetables you think you need to supplement your leftovers and add to the onion.

3. Add your leftovers, tomatoes, seasoning and stock. Bring to a simmer.

4. Add the pasta and cook until the pasta is to your liking. If you have some fresh or frozen herbs add them now.

5. Serve with crusty, multi-grain bread.

This is a quick way to make another meal with leftover sauces. There are lots of ways to adapt the recipe:

- Instead of macaroni try orzo pasta or use up leftover rice.

- Use up stale bread by breaking it into the bottom of the serving bowl with some crumbled cheese (a small amount of blue cheese is particularly good) and ladle the hot soup on top.

- Extend the soup further, by adding a can of beans, chickpeas or lentils (leftover lentils prepared for the Lentil and Tomato salad could be added).

Canned and frozen foods are often seen as a poorer choice than fresh. However, they are often similar in nutritional content or may even be higher than in fresh. Canned foods may have salt or sugar added so it is worth checking labels. As canned and frozen foods have a longer shelf-life, they are often cheaper, so help to keep food costs down and reduce food waste.

Lamb Tagine

Ready in **1 hour 30 minutes** • Serves **6**

Slow cooked casseroles are truly comfort food. Making use of a slow cooker can mean a hot bowl of something delicious at the end of a busy day – simply serve and eat. This can be very helpful when everyone in the house needs to eat at different times. Using a slow cooker is one of lowest cost cooking methods too, with no sacrifice on the taste of a dish like this.

Tagine has a wonderful flavour with a delicate blend of spices. Dried fruit and chickpeas add fibre, micronutrients and extra variety of plant foods in this dish. They also help to extend the meat, making the meal go further. It also means that this red meat dish is low in saturated fat which may be surprising. If you like a bit of spice, look for some harissa to add some heat.

Nutrition per serving:

340 cals • 12 g fat (2.7 g saturates) • 33 g carbs (20 g total sugars)
12 g fibre • 19 g protein • 0.4 g salt

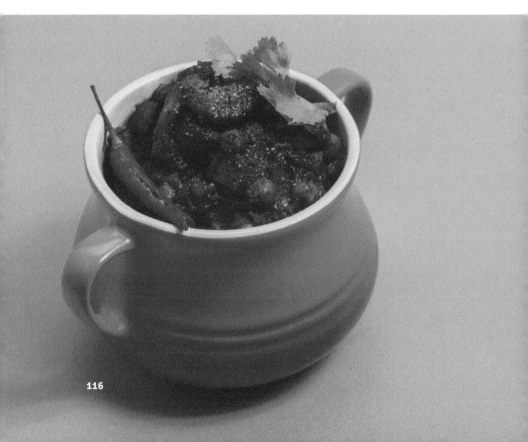

Ingredients

2 tbsp olive oil

300 g diced lamb

1 large onion, diced

2 medium carrots, diced

2 garlic cloves, finely chopped

2 tbsp ras-el-hanut or a mix of cinnamon, cumin, turmeric and black pepper

800 g canned tomatoes

800 g canned chickpeas, drained

100 g dried apricots

300 mls stock

Preparation

1. Heat the oven to 180 °C/fan 160 °C/gas mark 4 or have your slow cooker ready.

2. In a pot suitable to go in the oven, heat the olive oil and then add onions to gently cook.

3. When the onions are beginning to look translucent, add the lamb and brown on all sides.

4. Add the garlic and spices. Cook for about a minute, coating the meat and onions in the spices.

5. Add the carrots, tomatoes, chickpeas, apricots and stock to the pot, then bring to a simmer.

6. Put in the oven and cook for about an hour until the lamb is tender and flaking. You may need a little longer.

7. If using a slow cooker, after step 5 tip into your slow cooker and select the setting that you require according to your cooker.

8. Smell the aromas while it cooks and serve with flatbreads warmed in the oven or wholemeal couscous.

Swap lamb for chicken thighs (remove the skin) or cheaper cuts of beef that are intended for long slow cooking.

Make it vegetarian by adding extra chickpeas and more vegetables such as sweet potatoes, peppers, courgettes, green beans etc.

Make plenty as it's great for a leftover lunch - perfect over a jacket potato or with crusty bread.

Extend the leftovers for another meal - it's the perfect base for our Magic Minestrone for example.

Instant couscous

- Measure half a cup (about 90g) of couscous per person into a bowl (wholemeal couscous adds more fibre).

- Add flavour - a quarter teaspoon of stock powder per person and your preferred herbs and spices. Try ras-el-hanut and freshly ground black pepper.

- Add some raisins or finely chopped apricots.

- Mix in double the volume of boiling water, cover, and leave to stand for 5 minutes. The water should be absorbed and the couscous soft. You may need a little extra boiling water.

Any leftovers can be turned into a salad. Add finely chopped spring or red onions, tomatoes, some feta cheese or leftover roast meat or some chopped nuts, then a little dressing of your choice.

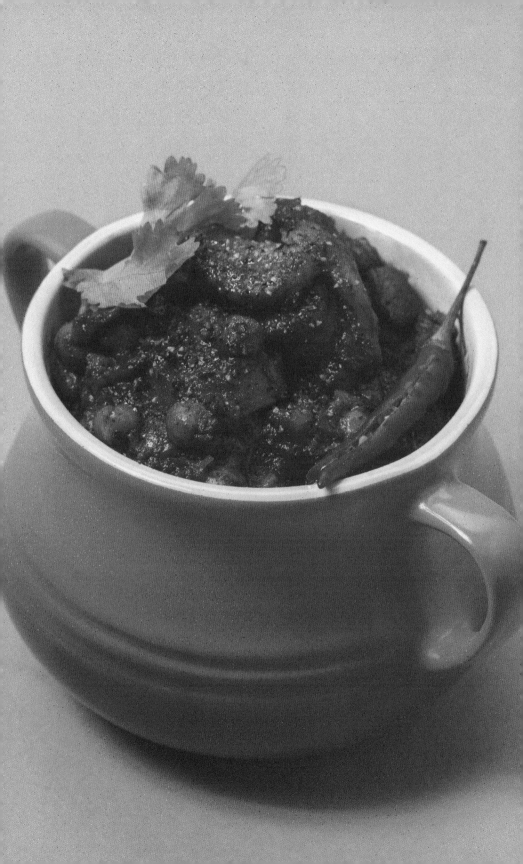

Kerala Style Chicken Curry

Ready in **40 minutes** • Serves **6**

A curry inspired by flavours of Kerala in India. Although there is a long list of ingredients it is worth it and the recipe is straightforward. Some women find spicy food exacerbates their hot flushes although it is very personal. The beauty of making your own curry rather than using a shop bought paste or a ready meal allows you to choose the spices to suit you.

Nutrition per serving:

357 cals • 12 g fat (5.1 g saturates) • 20 g carbs (8.5 g total sugars)

5.5 g fibre • 38 g protein • 0.4 g salt

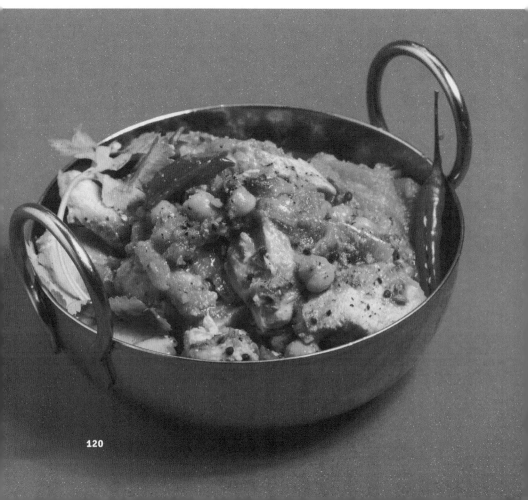

Ingredients

Spice paste

Ginger – a thumb sized piece

7 large cloves of garlic

1 tsp brown mustard seeds

1 tsp cumin seeds

½ tsp turmeric

2 tsps fennel seeds

1 tsp garam masala (optional)

½ tsp black peppercorns

Chilli (optional)

Curry ingredients

2 tbsp rapeseed/canola oil

1 large onion, sliced

750 g chicken – chicken thighs or legs cook well or chicken breasts (remove the skin)

1 small sweet potato, diced

400 g can chickpeas

1 pepper, diced (any colour)

2 large tomatoes, pureed

400 mls light coconut milk

Chopped coriander (optional)

Preparation

1. Start by making the spice paste. Using a blender whizz the garlic and ginger with about 100 mls of water until it is a puree. Then add all the spices and whizz again.

2. Fry the onion in the oil until they are soft and beginning to colour. Add your spice mix to the onions and fry to reduce it to a paste – about two minutes.

3. Add your chicken and stir for a couple of minutes to slightly brown and cover in the spices.

4. If you are making a vegetarian version add extra vegetables such as a diced aubergine, a handful of button mushrooms etc.

5. Throw in your vegetables and then add about 200 mls of water and the tomatoes. Cover and simmer on a low heat for about 20 minutes, stirring occasionally. There should be lots of sauce which will need thickening so increase the heat and remove the lid to allow the sauce to reduce.

6. When the sauce is thicker, add the coconut milk. If you have some coriander whether fresh or frozen, it can be added at this point. Heat the curry back up to a gentle simmer for a few minutes and then you are ready to serve.

7. Serve with rice or Indian breads and chutneys.

Serve with brown rice to add more fibre and a nuttier, chewier texture.

Leftover curry is delicious in a wrap or tortilla for lunch.

Lower the saturated fat, by leaving out the coconut milk. For a creamy finish, add some plain yoghurt or soya cream at the end of cooking.

Double the quantities of ingredients for the spice blend and store the paste in a jar to use another day.

Frozen ginger and garlic can be used for ease.

Use the spice paste to make a quick and tasty noodle soup.

Add about a tablespoon of paste to approximately 300 mls of water, bring to the boil and add a block of noodles with some diced vegetables (fresh, frozen or canned), leftover meat or cubes of tofu. Add a splash of soya sauce or sweet chilli sauce and you have a delicious and quick lunch.

Herbs and spices are one of the richest sources of a group of plant chemicals called polyphenols. In the large intestine, these chemicals help increase beneficial bacteria such as *Bifidobacterium* and *Lactobacillus*. These strains provide anti-pathogenic and anti-inflammatory effects.

Herbs and spices count towards the variety of plants in your diet even though they are only eaten in small amounts. Because they also add so much flavour they can help us to use less salt. Many of us eat more than the recommended maximum of 6 g of salt per day. So reach for the herbs and spices rather than the salt.

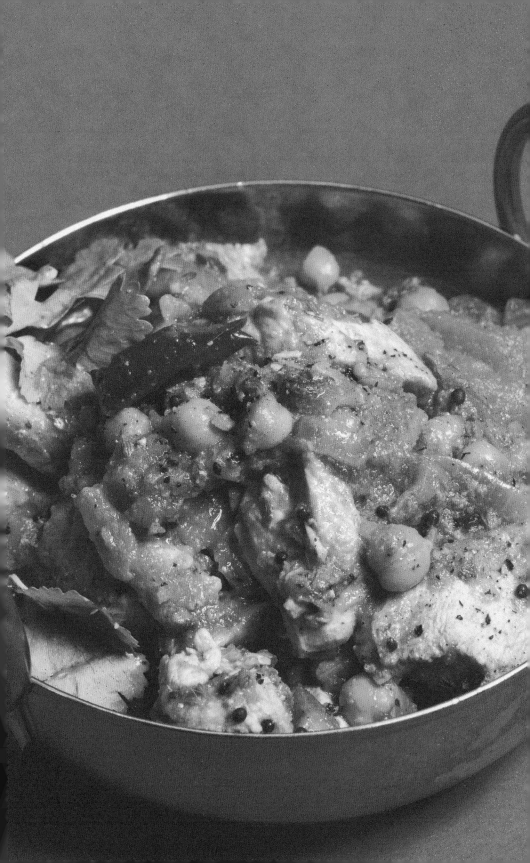

Salmon with Pesto Crust

Ready in **30 minutes** • Serves **6**

This is a simple recipe to give you a portion of oily fish with beneficial omega-3 fatty acids and vitamin D, with pesto to add a real blast of colour and flavour. The crunchy crust adds some texture and fibre, and the seeds also add a little omega-3 fats and a variety of vitamins and minerals.

Serve with green vegetables and new potatoes or mash. You could also serve it with our Lentil and Tomato Salad for a protein-filled meal.

Nutrition per serving (with new potatoes and spinach):

366 cals • 19 g fat (3.5 g saturates) • 21 g carbs (1.7 g total sugars)
3.9 g fibre • 25 g protein • 0.3 g salt

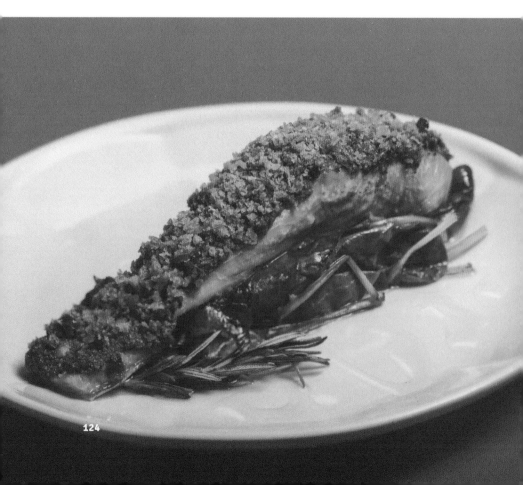

Ingredients

6 small fillets of salmon (about 500-600 g)

2-3 tbsp of your favourite pesto - this recipe uses the walnut pesto recipe below

2 slices of wholemeal/granary or seeded bread

1-2 tbsp mixed seeds of your choice

350 g of spinach

700 g new potatoes

Preparation

1. Heat the oven to 230 °C/fan 210 °C/gas 8.

2. Spread the pesto over the tops of the salmon fillets.

3. Turn your bread into fine breadcrumbs (using a food processor or grater) and mix with the mixed seeds.

4. Stick the crumb mix on top of the pesto and cook for 10-15 minutes until the salmon is cooked and the crumb is golden.

5. Serve on a bed of wilted spinach with steamed new potatoes.

Try this recipe with trout, which is another oily fish, or with white fish such as hake or coley.

Compare the label of ready-made pesto jars as some can be very high in salt. It's easy to make your own pesto - see below.

Spinach and Walnut Pesto

There are many recipes for regular basil pesto however many different green leaves and nuts can be used. This recipe uses spinach but any bagged leaves could be used like watercress or rocket. You could swap walnuts for pine nuts or cashew nuts.

- In a food processor or blender, whizz 160 g of spinach, 50 g of walnuts, 2-3 cloves of garlic, 30 g of grated parmesan or similar Italian cheese and 120 mls of olive oil or cold-pressed rapeseed oil.

- Add a squeeze of lemon juice and freshly ground black pepper.

The pesto can be stored for a few days in the fridge, or freeze in an ice cube tray for another day.

Salmon is rich in tryptophan, an amino acid that helps the body produce serotonin and melatonin, which can help with sleep. Low Vitamin D levels may be linked with poorer sleep quality. Salmon and other oily fish are one of the few dietary sources of vitamin D.

Lentil Shepherd's Pie

Ready in **1 hour 30 minutes** • Serves **6**

This traditional dish comes with a secret ingredient - lentils. Lentils add flavour and texture along with fibre, protein and micronutrients.

If you are looking to eat less red meat but have some resistance from other members of the household then this is a good recipe to try, particularly if you half the amount of meat in your regular recipe and top up with lentils.

Puy or other dark lentils hold their shape well and give a meatier colour and taste to the sauce compared to other beans or lentils.

The mash topping, hiding your secret ingredient, also adds in a bit of extra plant variety with celeriac and sweet potato, bringing additional colour and flavour to the dish.

Nutrition per serving:

427 cals • 7.4 g fat (2.5 g saturates) • 66 g carbs (12 g total sugars)

12 g fibre • 18 g protein • 0.5 g salt

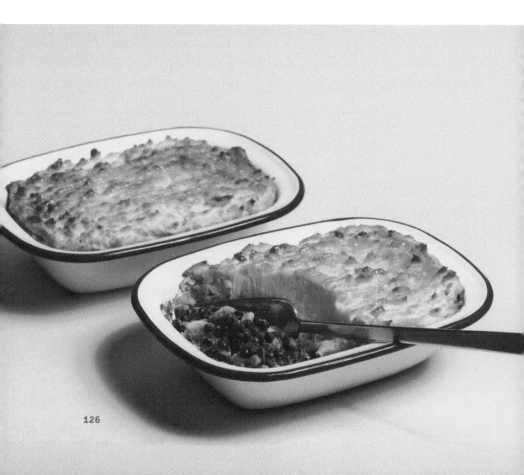

Ingredients

Filling:

1 tsp oil (olive or rapeseed/canola)

2 onions, chopped

2 cloves garlic (crushed or finely chopped)

2 tsp tomato puree

2 carrots, chopped

300 g Puy or other dried green lentils

1 tsp vegetable stock powder

Herbs de Provence or other dried herbs

Splash of dark soya sauce

750 mls water

Black pepper to your taste

Either cornflour or gravy granules to thicken the gravy to your liking.

Handful of frozen peas

Topping:

2 large potatoes, peeled and cut into medium-sized chunks

Half a celeriac, peeled and cut into medium-sized chunks

1 sweet potato, peeled and cut into medium-sized chunks

Small knob butter (about 15 g)

30 mls milk

30 g grated cheese

Preparation

1. Sauté the onion in the oil until soft. Add the garlic and continue to heat for a minute.

2. Add the tomato puree and allow to cook for a minute.

3. Add the carrots, peas and any other vegetables you wish to along with the stock, lentils and herbs.

4. Allow to simmer until the lentils are cooked. You may need to add extra water if the lentils absorb a lot of water.

5. While your lentils simmer, cook your potatoes, celeriac and sweet potato in boiling water until tender. Mash well with a little butter.

6. Thicken the lentil gravy sauce to your liking and spoon into an oven-proof dish. Top it with the mash and sprinkle with a little cheese.

7. Put under a hot grill to get a golden top. This can be made in advance and then put into a preheated oven 190 °C/fan 170 °C/gas mark 5 for about 30-40 minutes until piping hot throughout and a golden topping. Serve with steamed vegetables.

Ready cooked lentils from a can or pouch could be used - add less water, similar to when cooking minced beef in a gravy.

Reduce the amount of meat in a regular Shepherd's pie by replacing half the quantity of meat with lentils - it still tastes meaty but adds fibre to your meal.

To add an alternative plant protein, replace half the lentils with soya mince or mycoprotein.

Vary the mash with any root vegetables or stick to traditional mashed potato. Make extra mash to use for making fish cakes on another day.

This meal is a perfect batch cook recipe. Individual portions can be frozen to provide homemade ready meals.

Canned fish mixed with leftover mashed potato is the basis of healthy fishcakes.

Mix together: finely chopped spring onions, mashed potato, and a can of fish (e.g. tuna, salmon or sardines). Coat balls of the mixture in breadcrumbs with seeds added if you like. Flatten them, place on a baking tray and cook in the oven until piping hot and golden in colour.

Mycoprotein and soya mince are useful high quality plant substitutes for meat that can help reduce saturated fat and add fibre.

Mycoprotein, available as mince, nuggets and sausages, is made from a natural fungus called *Fusaraium venenatum*. The fungus is fermented to promote the growth of the mycoprotein.

Soya mince, chunks or sausages are versatile products to replace meat. These products provide phytoestrogens which may help manage hot flushes. Soya protein can also help lower cholesterol. Some soya products can be high in salt so check the labels.

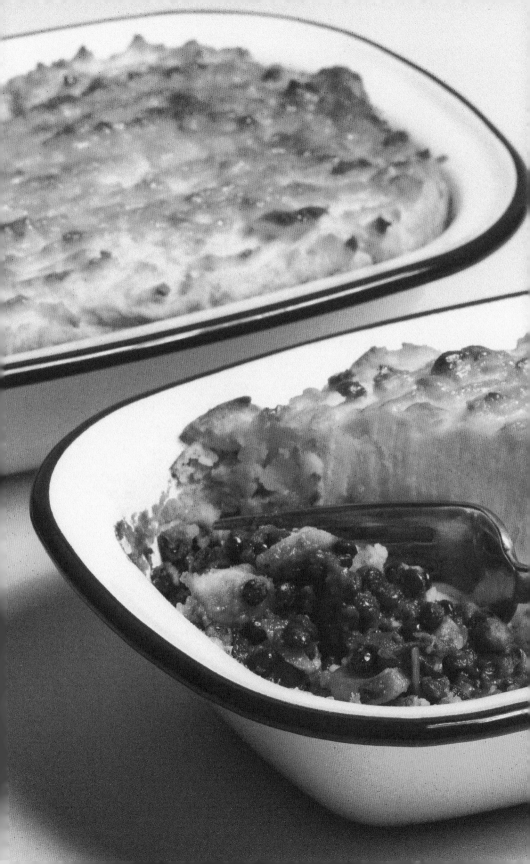

Tofu Satay Stir-fry & Noodles

Ready in **30 minutes** • Serves **4**

Tofu is a staple in many South-East Asian cuisines and is a rich source of phytoestrogens. If you are a tofu novice then this simple stir-fry is a good introduction. When buying tofu for this recipe, you will need firm tofu. Some varieties will need to be squeezed and drained, others are ready to use so check the pack for instructions.

Pick a mixture of vegetables to stir-fry - maybe what you have in the fridge or a pack of fresh or frozen stir-fry vegetables. If you want something a little different try Pak choi, tenderstem broccoli, mangetout and baby sweetcorn. There is no right or wrong.

Nutrition per serving (when served with soba noodles):

392 cals • 16 g fat (3.8 g saturates) • 30 g carbs (5.4 g total sugars)

7.8 g fibre • 28 g protein • 1 g salt

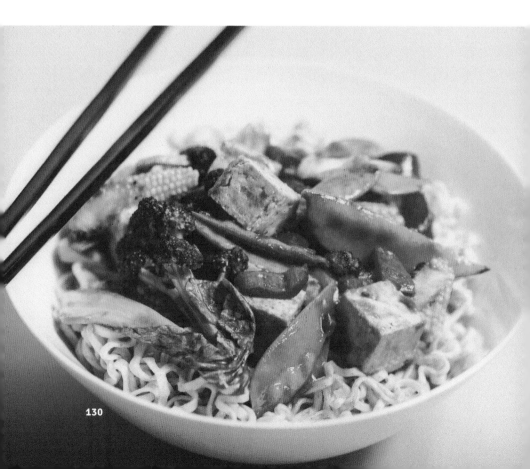

Ingredients

280 g firm tofu (a standard pack), marinated in reduced salt soy sauce, ginger, garlic, a little oil and chilli if desired

500 g vegetables to stir-fry

A clove of garlic

Thumb-size piece of ginger

4 or 5 spring onions

200 g soba noodles (or try wholewheat noodles)

1 tbsp rapeseed/canola oil (for frying)

Satay Sauce

1 tbsp reduced salt soy sauce (you could use the marinade)

1 tsp Chinese 5 spice

2 tbsp peanut butter

200 mls boiling water

Chilli (optional)

Preparation

1. Marinate the tofu for at about an hour. Or you can use pre-marinated or smoked tofu.

2. Put some rapeseed oil in a frying pan or wok and stir-fry your marinated tofu until golden and set aside.

3. Prepare about 500 g of vegetables - choose what you have in your fridge or your favourites. Onions or spring onions, broccoli, Pak choi, cabbage, peppers, mushrooms, carrots in thin strips, mangetout, baby sweetcorn, green beans, courgette...whatever you like. You could also use a pack of pre-prepared fresh or frozen stir-fried vegetables.

4. Peel and finely chop some garlic and ginger - you can use frozen or puree from a jar instead if you prefer.

5. Prepare your satay sauce: In a mug, mix the peanut butter, reduced salt soy sauce, Chinese 5 Spice and some sweet chilli (or other chilli if you like some heat). Add about 200 ml boiling water and mix to form a smooth sauce.

6. Stir-fry your vegetables on a high heat for 5 minutes or until tender. Add the tofu and satay sauce and mix thoroughly.

7. Boil some water and cook the noodles according to packet instructions whilst you are stir frying your vegetables.

8. Pile the stir-fry on top of the cooked noodles, or mix them together if you prefer.

9. Alternatively, you could serve the stir-fry with rice.

Tofu and peanut butter are rich in protein and other nutrients. Good additions if you are choosing to eat less or no animal foods.

Choose firm tofu that is set using calcium, particularly if you exclude dairy products.

Wholewheat noodles are a good source of fibre.

Leftovers make a tasty noodle salad, or use the stir-fry vegetables in a wrap for lunch.

Adding lots of soya in a short time may upset your stomach at first. If soya is a new food for you, add it gradually.

Peanuts are not true nuts. They are a legume rich in protein and similar to tree nuts in nutritional value.

Both peanuts and tree nuts have been shown to be beneficial for health but are often avoided as they are high in fat. However, they provide healthy fats, fibre and a range of nutrients that are beneficial for heart health.

Peanut and other nut butters are versatile ingredients which can help add protein through the day. As a toast topping, stirred into porridge or a smoothie at breakfast, as a sandwich filling or in a sauce, adding protein to a vegetarian dish.

Check labels on jars of nut butters as they can have salt, sugar and less healthy fats added to them.

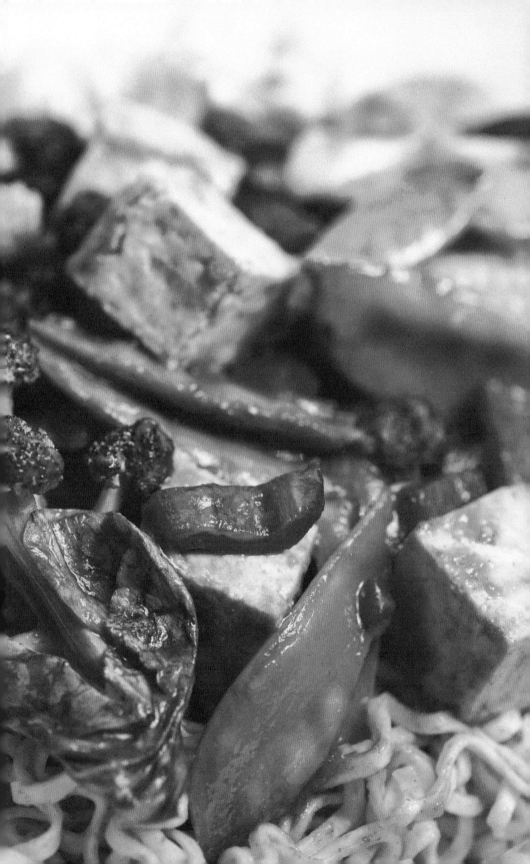

Chocolate Hummus

Ready in **15-20 minutes** • Serves **8**

It sounds bizarre but give it a go!

This snack gives you a chocolate hit and provides both protein and fibre. It's perfect to spread on crackers or to dip fruit into. For something more dessert like, spoon over summer fruit coulis made simply by defrosting frozen summer fruits and berries.

Nutrition per serving:

87 cals • 2.7 g fat (0.6 g saturates) • 7.8 g carbs (3.1 g total sugars)
1.9 g fibre • 6.8 g protein • 0.2 g salt

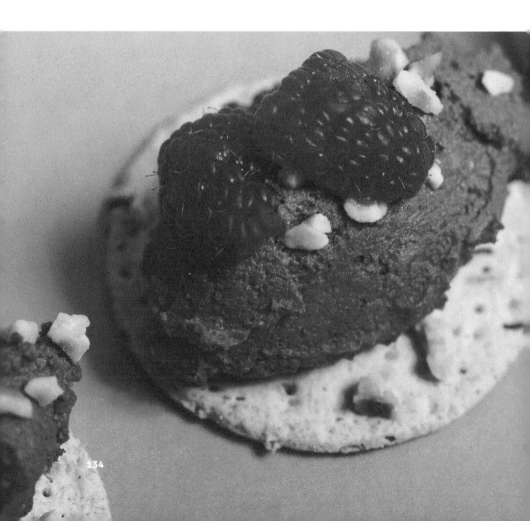

Ingredients

400 g chickpeas, drained and rinsed.

1 tbsp tahini paste

3-4 tbsp cocoa powder

2-3 tbsp Maple syrup or similar (to your taste to balance the bitter cocoa) or use soft brown sugar

1 tbsp water or milk/milk alternative

Preparation

1. Put all the ingredients except the liquid into a food processor or blender and whizz until smooth. Add water or milk or milk alternative of your choice to get the consistency you prefer.

2. Add extras for additional flavour and texture such as nuts, seeds, chocolate chips, vanilla extract or berries.

Raspberries, fresh or frozen, or a squeeze of orange juice adds a fruity tang.

Swap the tahini for a nut butter. Hazelnut butter or ground hazelnuts are particularly good.

Stir in dark chocolate chips and warm in the microwave for a pudding with oozy chocolate mouthfuls.

Chickpeas are very versatile. Rich in protein and micronutrients, they can be added to soups, sauces and stews; blended to make hummus; or made into falafel-style fritters. Roasted chickpeas, seasoned with spices, make a tasty, protein-rich snack.

Dried chickpeas can be ground into gram flour. Gluten-free and rich in protein, it can be used to thicken sauces, made into pancakes or used in baking.

The protein-rich water from canned chickpeas, known as aquafaba, can be used in place of eggs for baking or to make meringues.

Oaty Apple Muffins

Ready in **35 minutes** • Makes about **10-12 muffins**

Muffins are quick to make. They don't need much butter, egg or sugar, but are moist and tasty. These ones are a great breakfast on-the-go, with the oats providing fibre which can help you feel full for longer. Lovely warm from the oven or reheat them in the microwave for a few seconds.

Nutrition per muffin (if 12 are made):

144 cals • 5.1 g fat (1.9 g saturates) • 21 g carbs (9.3 g total sugars)

1.6 g fibre • 2.8 g protein • 0.4 g salt

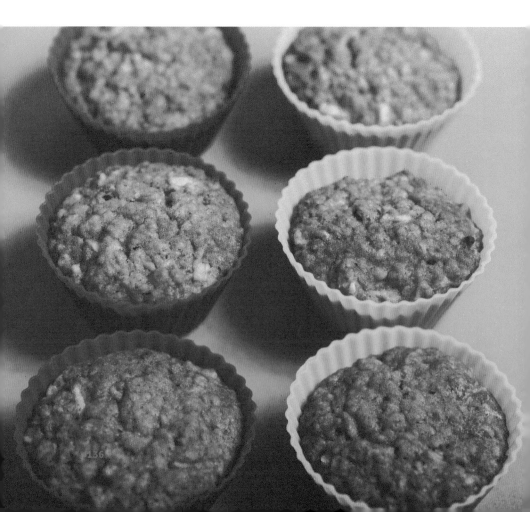

Ingredients

125 g self-raising flour

80 g oats

90 g soft brown sugar

2 tsp ground cinnamon

1 level tsp bicarbonate soda

75 g butter or 60 % fat spread/
butter

1 egg, lightly beaten

1 medium apple, peeled and
grated

60 mls milk

Preparation

1. Preheat the oven to 200 °C/fan 180 °C/gas mark 6.

2. Measure the dry ingredients into a bowl and mix well.

3. Melt the butter then add the wet ingredients including the grated apple.

4. Mix the wet ingredients with the dry ingredients until the flour is just mixed in - do not overmix. It is fine for the mixture to be a bit lumpy.

5. Divide the mixture into muffin cases and bake for 12- 15 minutes. They should be golden and spring back when pressed.

When mixing the ingredients, less is better - they won't be so light if you mix the batter too much.

Swap butter for 60 % fat spread or reduced-fat butter for baking. The recipe still works and you lower the saturated fat.

Swap half the flour for wholemeal self-raising flour to add some extra fibre. You could also add a few tablespoons of dried fruit or seeds to the dry ingredients.

The muffins freeze well and can be defrosted overnight to be warmed for breakfast.

When we compare muffins made like these with a homemade, plain sponge cake, muffins are almost half the calories (per 100 g), have less than half the fat and 10 g less sugar. This recipe also has three times the amount of fibre per 100 g. These muffins are a better and healthier bake than regular cupcakes.

Amazeballs

Ready in **15-20 minutes** • Makes about **15-20**, easy to scale up

These are amazing - sweet but not overly so, and adaptable with different flavour options. The almonds provide protein, the dates sweetness and fibre, and oats have soluble fibre that has beneficial effects on cholesterol. They also pass the child/teenager test!

Approximate nutrition per ball (If twenty balls are made) :

56 cals • 2.5 g fat (0.2 g saturates) • 6.5 g carbs (4.7 g total sugars)
1 g fibre • 1.5 g protein • 0 g salt

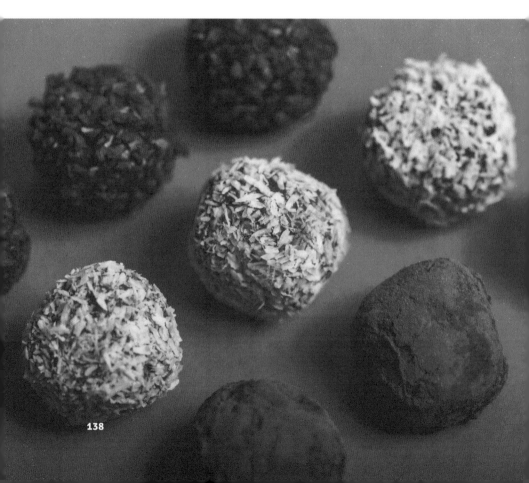

Ingredients

14 dates, stone removed

6 tbsp ground almonds

Splash of water

4 tbsp oats

Optional flavours -

cocoa powder (1-2 tbsp)

Replace 1-2 tbsp ground almonds with the same of desiccated coconut

orange zest (add to your taste)

chopped dried cranberries (works well with orange zest)

mixed spice for a Christmas taste

Grated carrot and ground ginger

Cocoa and chopped crystallised ginger

Preparation

1. Put the pitted dates and ground almonds into a food processor or the processor fitting on a handheld blender with a splash of water. If you add more water, you will get a softer, ganache-like texture.

2. When you have a sticky mixture that is blended well, add the oats and whizz again. You can add your optional flavours here or mix them in after. Spices and cocoa can be added here, if you want bits of cranberry/orange zest/carrot noticeable in the final balls then mix in afterwards.

3. When you have a mixture that you can form easily into balls then tip it into a bowl, add any additions that give texture as well as taste and mix them in.

4. If you want, you can roll the balls in a range of things: cocoa powder, icing sugar, desiccated coconut, chopped nuts, vermicelli (sprinkles), freeze-dried chopped raspberries, toasted seeds, sesame seeds...you get the idea. Be creative!

These are a satisfying sweet snack. The dates provide all the sweetness and combined with the other ingredients, provide protein, fibre and micronutrients.

The basic recipe is easy to adjust with different flavours. The nutrient content is very approximate as it depends on their size and what additions you use.

Do check whether the dates you use are pitted or not before throwing them in your blender. It seems obvious but an easy thing to forget.

Roll them in cocoa powder, desiccated coconut or dried raspberries - they look so good and make a lovely gift.

Oaty Berry Squares

Ready in **30 minutes** • Makes **16 slices**

These tasty and satisfying squares are made with only a few ingredients, so they are super straightforward to do. They are high in fibre and micronutrients such as magnesium and phosphorous which are important for maintaining bone health. They also provide a range of vitamins and minerals that help support brain function and mood, and of course they sweet and delicious!

Nutrition per square:

155 cals • 5.1 g fat (1.4 g saturates) • 21 g carbs (6.5 g total sugars)

4 g fibre • 4.2 g protein • 0 g salt

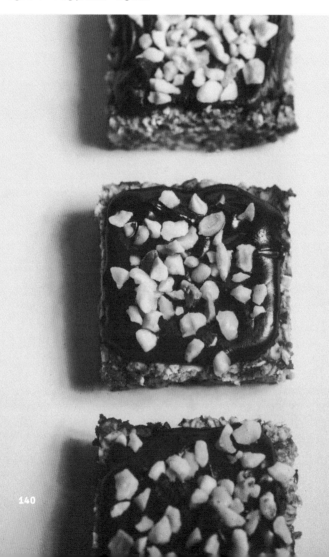

Ingredients

350 g rolled oats

50 g flaxseeds

200 ml soya milk alternative (or dairy milk)

200 g raspberries (fresh or frozen)

75 g soft brown sugar

About 60 g dark chocolate for melting on top

Preparation

1. Heat the oven to 200 °C/fan 180 °C/gas mark 6.

2. In a bowl, mix the oats, flaxseeds and soya milk alternative until its combined and the mix is quite stiff.

3. Add in the sugar and berries and mix thoroughly. Don't worry if some of the berries get squashed.

4. Put the mixture into the baking tin (23 cm by 23 cm or a similar size) and flatten down with the back of a spoon.

5. Bake for 25-30 minutes until the top turns golden and feels quite firm if you press down in the middle.

6. Leave to cool for 10 minutes.

7. Melt the chocolate in a microwave – heat in a microwave for about 40 seconds, taking it out regularly and stirring so it doesn't over heat. Pour roughly over the squares.

8. Cut into 16 squares. These keep well for a few days if stored in an airtight container.

Press the mixture firmly into the tray so the squares hold together well.

Swap raspberries for other fruit like blueberries, blackberries or cherries. You could use frozen mixed fruit.

Drizzle almond butter on top either instead of, or along with the chocolate. Top with a sprinkle of crushed nuts or seeds for added crunch.

These are delicious served warm or cold.

Oats are a good source of fibre. Particularly rich in a soluble fibre called beta-glucan, adding oats to your day can benefit heart health. By forming a gel in the gut, beta-glucan combines with cholesterol to reduce its absorption, helping to maintain healthy cholesterol levels.

Just 3 servings of oat-based foods a day can provide the optimum 3 g of beta-glucan for lowering cholesterol. An oaty snack like this is a delicious and satisfying way to add beta-glucan to your day.

References

Introduction

British Menopause Society (2017) New survey highlights impact of the menopause on every aspect of women's lives in the UK. https://thebms.org.uk/2017/10/world-menopause-day-2/

The Menopause Management (2022) Transgender—LGBTQIA+ people experiencing the menopause. https://themenopausemanagement.co.uk/lgbtqia/

Hot Flushes

Messina, M., Mejia, S. B et al. (2022) Neither soy foods nor isoflavones warrant classification as endocrine disruptors: A technical review of the observational and clinical data. Critical Reviews in Food Science and Nutrition, 62(21), 5824–5885. https://doi.org/10.1080/10408398.2021.1895054

Rock My Menopause (2022) Symptoms. https://rockmymenopause.com/get-informed/symptoms/

Taku, K., Melby, M. K et al. (2021) Extracted or synthesized soybean isoflavones reduce menopausal hot flash frequency and severity: Systematic review and meta-analysis of randomized controlled trials. Menopause, 19(7), 776–790.

Healthy Weight Management

Best, N., & Flannery, O (2023) Association between adherence to the Mediterranean Diet and the Eatwell Guide and changes in weight and waist circumference in post-menopausal women in the UK Women's Cohort Study. Post Reproductive Health, 29(1), 25–32. https://doi.org/10.1177/20533691231156643

Gibson, S., & Ashwell, M (2020) A simple cut-off for waist-to-height ratio (0·5) can act as an indicator for cardiometabolic risk: Recent data from adults in the Health Survey for England. British Journal of Nutrition, 123(6), 681–690. https://doi.org/10.1017/S0007114519003301

Mamerow, M. M., Mettler, J. A et al. (2014) Dietary Protein Distribution Positively Influences 24-h Muscle Protein Synthesis in Healthy Adults. The Journal of Nutrition, 144(6), 876–880. https://doi.org/10.3945/jn.113.185280

Marlatt, K. L., Pitynski-Miller, D. R. et al. (2022) Body composition and cardiometabolic health across the menopause transition. Obesity, 30(1), 14–27. https://doi.org/10.1002/oby.23289

PHE (Public Health England) (2018) The Eatwell Guide. https://www.gov.uk/government/publications/the-eatwell-guide

Heart Health

Action on Salt, Action on Sugar & The George Institute for Global Health (2022) FoodSwitch UK. http://www.foodswitch.co.uk/

Aune, D., Giovannucci, E et al. (2017) Fruit and vegetable intake and the risk of cardiovascular disease, total cancer and all-cause mortality—A systematic review and dose-response meta-analysis of prospective studies. International Journal of Epidemiology, 46(3), 1029–1056. https://doi.org/10.1093/ije/dyw319

Aune, D., Keum, N et al. (2016) Whole grain consumption and risk of cardiovascular disease, cancer, and all cause and cause specific mortality: Systematic review and dose-response meta-analysis of prospective studies. BMJ, i2716. https://doi.org/10.1136/bmj.i2716

BHF (British Heart Foundation) (2022) BHF Statistics Factsheet—UK. https://www.bhf.org.uk/what-we-do/our-research/heart-statistics

Heart UK (2022) Top 7 things to know about using plant sterols and stanols to reduce blood cholesterol levels. https://www.heartuk.org.uk/healthy-living/flora-proactiv-2

Kim, Y., Keogh, J., & Clifton, P (2018) Nuts and Cardio-Metabolic Disease: A Review of Meta-Analyses. Nutrients, 10(12), 1935. https://doi.org/10.3390/nu10121935

Kou, T., Wang, Q et al. (2017) Effect of soybean protein on blood pressure in postmenopausal women: A meta-analysis of randomized controlled trials. Food & Function, 8(8), 2663–2671.

NHS (2021) Tips for a lower salt diet. https://www.nhs.uk/live-well/eat-well/how-to-eat-a-balanced-diet/tips-for-a-lower-salt-diet/

NHS (2022) NHS stop smoking services help you quit. https://www.nhs.uk/live-well/quit-smoking/nhs-stop-smoking-services-help-you-quit/

NHS Digital (2020) Health Survey for England 2019: Adults health report. https://digital.nhs.uk/data-and-information/publications/statistical/health-survey-for-england/2019

NICE (2022) Obesity: Identification, assessment and management [Clinical Guidance 189]. https://www.nice.org.uk/guidance/cg189/chapter/Recommendations

Public Health England (2016) Government Dietary Recommendations for energy and nutrients for males and females aged 1-18 years and 19+ years. https://assets.publishing.service.gov.uk/government/uploads/system/uploads/attachment_data/file/618167/government_dietary_recommendations.pdf

Ramdath, D., Padhi, E et al. (2017) Beyond the Cholesterol-Lowering Effect of Soy Protein: A Review of the Effects of Dietary Soy and Its Constituents on Risk Factors for Cardiovascular Disease. Nutrients, 9(4), 324. https://doi.org/10.3390/nu9040324

Reynolds, A., Mann, J et al. (2019) Carbohydrate quality and human health: A series of systematic reviews and meta-analyses. The Lancet, 393(10170), 434–445. https://doi.org/10.1016/S0140-6736(18)31809-9

Slopien, R., Wender-Ozegowska, E et al. (2018) Menopause and diabetes: EMAS clinical guide. Maturitas, 117, 6–10. https://doi.org/10.1016/j.maturitas.2018.08.009

Vogel, B., Acevedo, M et al. (2021) The Lancet women and cardiovascular disease Commission: Reducing the global burden by 2030. Lancet, 397(10292), 2385–2438.

Bone Health

British Dietetic Association (2019) Osteoporosis and diet: Food Fact Sheet. https://www.bda.uk.com/resource/osteoporosis-diet.html

Cardwell, G., Bornman, J. F et al. (2018) A Review of Mushrooms as a Potential Source of Dietary Vitamin D. Nutrients, 10(10), 1498.

Heaney, R. P., & Rafferty, K (2006) The Settling Problem in Calcium-Fortified Soybean Drinks. Journal of the American Dietetic Association, 106(11), 1753. https://doi.org/10.1016/j.jada.2006.08.008

Public Health England (2020) National Diet and Nutrition Survey. Rolling programme Years 9 to 11 (2016/2017 to 2018/2019) https://www.gov.uk/government/statistics/ndns-results-from-years-9-to-11-2016-to-2017-and-2018-to-2019

Royal Osteoporosis Society (2020) Key facts and statistics. https://theros.org.uk/what-we-do/media-centre/media-toolkit/

Tong, T. Y. N., Appleby, P. N et al. (2020) Vegetarian and vegan diets and risks of total and site-specific fractures: Results from the prospective EPIC-Oxford study. BMC Medicine, 18(1), 353. https://doi.org/10.1186/s12916-020-01815-3

Mood and Mental Health

Hybholt, M (2022) Psychological and social health outcomes of physical activity around menopause: A scoping review of research. Maturitas, 164, 88–97. https://doi.org/10.1016/j.maturitas.2022.07.014

Jacka, F. N., O'Neil, A et al. (2017) A randomised controlled trial of dietary improvement for adults with major depression (the 'SMILES' trial). BMC Medicine, 15(1), 23. https://doi.org/10.1186/s12916-017-0791-y

McDonald, D., Hyde, E et al. (2018) American Gut: An Open Platform for Citizen Science Microbiome Research. 3(3), 28. https://doi.org/10.1128/msystems.00031-18

NIH. (2022). Omega-3 Fatty Acids—Health Professional Fact Sheet. https://ods.od.nih.gov/factsheets/Omega3FattyAcids-HealthProfessional/

Shaffiei, F., Salari-Moghaddam, A et al. (2019) Adherence to the Mediterranean diet and risk of depression: A systematic review and updated meta-analysis of observational studies. Nutrition Reviews, 77(4), 230–239.

Sleeping Well

Akhavizadegan, H., Locke, J. A et al. (2018) A comprehensive review of adult enuresis. Can Urol Assoc J, 13(8), 282–287.

Gao, Q., Kou, T et al. (2018) The Association between Vitamin D Deficiency and Sleep Disorders: A Systematic Review and Meta-Analysis. Nutrients, 10(10), 1395. https://doi.org/10.3390/nu10101395

Harrison, E. G., Keating, J. L., & Morgan, P. E (2019) Non-pharmacological interventions for restless legs syndrome: A systematic review of randomised controlled trials. Disability and Rehabilitation, 41(17), 2006–2014.

Innes, K. E., Selfe, T. K et al. (2020) Effects of a 12-week yoga versus a 12-week educational film intervention on symptoms of restless legs syndrome and related outcomes: An exploratory randomized controlled trial. Journal of Clinical Sleep Medicine, 16(1), 13.

Jehan, S., Masters-Isarilov, A et al. (2015) Sleep Disorders in Postmenopausal Women. J Sleep Disord Ther, 4(5), 212.

Ji, X., Grandner, M. A., & Liu, J (2017) The relationship between micronutrient status and sleep patterns: A systematic review. Public Health Nutrition, 20(4), 687-701.

Lee, J., Han, Y et al. (2019) Sleep Disorders and Menopause. Journal of Menopausal Medicine, 25(2), 83. https://doi.org/10.6118/jmm.19192

Leslie, S. W., Sajjad, H., & Singh, S (2022) Nocturia. In StatPearls. StatPearls Publishing LLC. https://www.ncbi.nlm.nih.gov/books/NBK518987/

Majid, M. S., Ahmad, H. S et al. (2017) The effect of vitamin D supplement on the score and quality of sleep in 20–50 year-old people with sleep disorders compared with control group. Nutritional Neuroscience, 21(7). https://www.tandfonline.com/doi/full/10.1080/1028415X.2017.1317395?scroll=top&needAccess=true

Meng, X., Li, Y et al. (2017) Dietary Sources and Bioactivities of Melatonin. Nutrients, 9(4), 367. https://doi.org/10.3390/nu9040367

Pan, Z., Wen, S et al. (2022) Different regimens of menopausal hormone therapy for improving sleep quality: A systematic review and meta-analysis. Menopause, 29(5), 627–635. https://doi.org/10.1097/GME.0000000000001945

Scoditti, E., Tumolo, M. R., & Garbarino, S (2022) Mediterranean Diet on Sleep: A Health Alliance. Nutrients, 14(14), 2998. https://doi.org/10.3390/nu14142998

Wesstrom, J., Nilsson, S., Sundstrom-Poromaa, I., & Ulfberg, J (2008) Restless legs syndrome among women: Prevalence, co-morbidity and possible relationship to menopause. Climacteric, 11(5), 422–428.

Women and Equality Committee (2022) Menopause and the workplace survey results. House of Commons. https://committees.parliament.uk/publications/8995/documents/152634/default/

Women's Health Concern (2021) Menopause and insomnia. https://www.womens-health-concern.org/wp-content/uploads/2021/09/17-WHC-FACTSHEET-Menopause-and-insomnia-SEPT2021.pdf

Healthy Hydration

Benelam, B., & Wyness, L (2010) Hydration and health: A review. Nutrition Bulletin, 35(1), 3–25.

Healthy Hair, Skin and Eyes

Garcia-Alfaro, P., Bergamaschi, L et al. (2020) Prevalence of ocular surface disease symptoms in peri- and postmenopausal women. Menopause, 27(9), 993–998.

Liu, A., & Ji, J. (2014) Omega-3 Essential Fatty Acids Therapy for Dry Eye Syndrome: A Meta-Analysis of Randomized Controlled Studies. Medical Science Monitor, 20, 1583–1589. https://doi.org/10.12659/MSM.891364

Suri, V., & Suri, V (2014) Menopause and oral health. Journal of Mid-Life Health, 5(3), 115. https://doi.org/10.4103/0976-7800.141187

Zouboulis, C. C., Blume-Peytavi, U et al. (2022) Skin, hair and beyond: The impact of menopause. Climacteric, 25(5), 434–442. https://doi.org/10.1080/13697137.2022.2050206

Myths and Marketing

Cienfuegos, S., Corapi, S et al. (2022) Effect of Intermittent Fasting on Reproductive Hormone Levels in Females and Males: A Review of Human Trials. Nutrients, 14(11), 2343. https://doi.org/10.3390/nu14112343

de Miranda, R. B., Weimer, P., & Rossi, R. C (2021) Effects of hydrolyzed collagen supplementation on skin aging: A systematic review and meta-analysis. International Journal of Dermatology, 60(12), 1449–1461. https://doi.org/10.1111/ijd.15518

Garcia-Coronado, J. M., Martinez-Olvera, L., & Elizondo-Omana, R. E (2019) Effect of collagen supplementation on osteoarthritis symptoms: A meta-analysis of randomized placebo-controlled trials. Int Orthop, 43, 531-538. https://doi.org/10.1007/s00264-018-4211-5

Geller, S. E., & Studee, L (2007) Botanical and Dietary Supplements for Menopausal Symptoms: What Works, What Doesn't. J Womens Health, 22.

Kanadys, W., Baranska, A., Jedrych, M., et al. (2020) Effects of red clover (Trifolium pratense) isoflavones on the lipid profile of perimenopausal and postmenopausal women- A systematic review and meta-analysis. Maturitas, 132, 7–16.

König, D., Oesser, S., Scharla, S., et al. (2018) Specific Collagen Peptides Improve Bone Mineral Density and Bone Markers in Postmenopausal Women—A Randomized Controlled Study. Nutrients, 10(1), 97. https://doi.org/10.3390/nu10010097

Krutmann, J., Bouloc, A., Sore, G., et al. (2017) The skin aging exposome. Journal of Dermatological Science, 85, 152–161.

Lee, H. W., Ang, L., & Lee, M. S (2022) Using ginseng for menopausal women's health care: A systematic review of randomized placebo-controlled trials. Complementary Therapies in Clinical Practice, 48, 101615.

Messina, M., Duncan, A., Messina, V., et al. (2022) The health effects of soy: A reference guide for health professionals. Frontiers in Nutrition, 9(970364). https://www.frontiersin.org/articles/10.3389/fnut.2022.970364/full

MHRA (2022) Herbal medicines granted a traditional herbal registration: Guidance. https://www.gov.uk/government/publications/herbal-medicines-granted-a-traditional-herbal-registration-thr/herbal-medicines-granted-a-traditional-herbal-registration

Mohammady, M., Janani, L., et al. (2018) Effect of omega-3 supplements on vasomotor symptoms in menopausal women: A systematic review and meta-analysis. European Journal of Obstetrics and Gynecology and Reproductive Biology, 228, 295–302.

National Institute of Health (2020) Health Information—National Centre for Complementary and Integrative Health. https://www.nccih.nih.gov/health

Shaw, G., Lee-Barthel, A., Ross, M. L. R., et al. (2017) Vitamin C–enriched gelatin supplementation before intermittent activity augments collagen synthesis. Am J Clin Nutr, 105, 136–143.

Spiro, A., & Lockyer, S (2018) Nutraceuticals and skin appearance: Is there any evidence to support this growing trend? Nutrition Bulletin, 43(1), 10–45.

Suez, J., Cohen, Y., & Valdes-Mas, R (2022) Personalized microbiome-driven effects of non-nutritive sweeteners on human glucose tolerance. Cell, 185(18), 3307–3328.

Tong, T. Y. N., Appleby, P. N., Armstrong, M. E. G., et al. (2020) Vegetarian and vegan diets and risks of total and site-specific fractures: Results from the prospective EPIC-Oxford study. BMC Medicine, 18(1), 353. https://doi.org/10.1186/s12916-020-01815-3

Zdzieblik, D., Oesser, S., & König, D (2021) Specific Bioactive Collagen Peptides in Osteopenia and Osteoporosis: Long-Term Observation in Postmenopausal Women. Journal of Bone Metabolism, 28(3), 207–213. https://doi.org/10.11005/jbm.2021.28.3.207

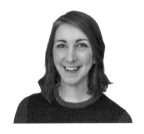

About Dr Laura Wyness

L aura is an award-winning Registered Nutritionist who specialises in nutrition writing, workplace wellness and nutrition communications.

With over 15-years' experience working in food innovation and academic research, Laura loves reviewing scientific evidence and translating it into clear messages.

She started working as a freelance Nutritionist in 2016 and was awarded 'Freelance Nutritionist of the Year' by the Caroline Walker Trust in 2019. Her nutrition consultancy work includes providing nutrition content, workplace wellness support and online nutrition consultations for individuals.

Laura has provided training for fellow health professionals on 'Menopause, Heart health and Cholesterol' (see MyNutriWeb.com). Before starting her freelance career, she worked at the Women's Health Council in Ireland, where her publication 'Managing Menopause' was awarded the Crystal-Clear Health Literacy Award.

Before championing healthy eating for menopause, Laura worked as a Senior Research Fellow in the Scottish Centre for Food Development and Innovation. She has appeared on TV and radio providing insight on various nutrition topics. One of her passions is helping connect people with healthy, local and sustainable food, which is the aim of her recent podcast 'Food Connections'.

Registered with the Association for Nutrition, Laura obtained a degree in Health Sciences and Nutrition, a Masters in Public Health and Health Services Research with distinction and a PhD whilst studying at the University of Aberdeen.

Follow Laura on Instagram @drlaurawyness, Twitter @laura_wyness and visit laurawyness.com.

Dr Laura Wyness

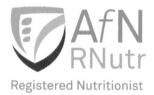

Registered Nutritionist

Protecting the public and promoting high standards in evidence-based science and professional practice of nutrition.

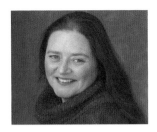

About Lynn Burns

Lynn Burns has been a Registered Nutritionist for more than 20 years.

Lynn began her career with the UK Government, which gave her a solid grounding in public health nutrition and sparked her interest in adapting nutrition messages to different groups for the most impact on health. Her work included nutrition analysis, science communication, managing Government-funded research on bone health and healthy ageing, and supporting advisory committees. She also worked on public consultations on nutrition and food allergy labelling and helped develop nutrition standards for food provided in care homes, workplace canteens, hospitals, and schools.

Lynn became a freelance nutritionist in 2011, spending several years as a Trustee for the Caroline Walker Trust, whose mission 'to improve public health through good food' and work on nutrition standards for specific groups has been a powerful influence. Recipe analysis and reformulation is a big part of Lynn's work. She has worked with school meal providers to improve meals, meet standards, and adapt menus for special dietary requirements. She regularly works with home economists and recipe developers and is responsible for the recipe analysis for 'Let's Talk Food 'projects.

Lynn also writes and delivers webinars and on-line courses for different groups including mothers, carers, people with long-term conditions such as Multiple Sclerosis and Parkinson's Disease, menopausal women, and fellow nutritionists.

In her spare time, Lynn volunteers as a Scout leader. She uses her experience to develop menus and cook nutritious food to fuel the adventurous activities of as many as 200 people at a time, with only a tent as a kitchen! She enjoys the opportunity to teach young people about food and nutrition.

Working with Laura on Eating Well for Menopause has been a timely adventure and Lynn now works directly with women approaching menopause, helping them improve their health through and beyond menopause with the food they eat.

Follow Lynn on Instagram @lynnburnsnutrition, on Twitter @LynnBurnsRNutr or lynnburnsnutrition.com

Printed in Great Britain
by Amazon

29852001R10089